Clinical Oral M

Clinical Oral Medicine

Michael A O Lewis, PhD, BDS, FDS, RCPS
Lecturer in Oral Medicine, Department of Oral Surgery, Medicine and Pathology,
University of Wales College of Medicine, Cardiff

and

Philip-John Lamey, BSc, BDS, MB, ChB, DDS, FDS, RCPS, FFD, RCSI
Professor of Oral Medicine, Queen's University, Belfast

Foreword by
Professor Sir David Mason
Glasgow Dental Hospital and School

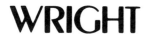

Wright
An imprint of Butterworth-Heinemann Ltd
Linacre House, Jordan Hill, Oxford OX2 8DP

R A member of the Reed Elsevier plc group

OXFORD   LONDON   BOSTON
MUNICH   NEW DELHI   SINGAPORE   SYDNEY
TOKYO   TORONTO   WELLINGTON

First published 1993
Reprinted 1995

British Library Cataloguing in Publication Data
Lewis, Michael A. O.
  Clinical Oral Medicine
  I. Title II. Lamey, Philip-John
  616.31

ISBN 0 7236 2255 8

Library of Congress Cataloguing in Publication Data
Lewis, Michael A. O.
  Clinical oral medicine/Michael A. O. Lewis and Philip-John Lamey.
  p.   cm.
  Includes bibliographical references and index.
  ISBN 0 7236 2255 8
  1. Oral medicine. I. Lamey, Philip-John. II. Title.
  [DNLM: 1. Stomatognathic Diseases – diagnosis. 2. Stomatognathic
  Diseases – therapy. WU 140 L675c 1993]
  RC815.L48 1993   93–20528
  617.5'22–dc20   CIP

Composition by Genesis Typesetting, Laser Quay, Rochester, Kent
Printed and bound in Great Britain by the Bath Press, Avon

Contents

Foreword

It gives me great pleasure to welcome a new book on Clinical Oral Medicine by two former colleagues.

Although the major part of the dentist's work is still of a restorative nature, the increasing involvement in prevention, diagnosis and treatment of oral diseases and the oral manifestation of systemic disease is becoming well recognized internationally.

The dentist's role has therefore been broadened to include the management of patients with soft tissue diseases such as oral cancer, and AIDS, facial pain, temporomandibular joint disorders and salivary dysfunction. In this way dental and oral health is increasingly being seen as part of general health. In such circumstances the need for the dentist to have more of an oral physician's approach and to be more concerned with the patient's previous history, drug history and lifestyle is obvious. This basic philosophy is emphasized throughout this book.

There is clearly a need for fundamental change in the education of the dentist and the dental team to accompany these changes in clincal practice reflecting the broader clinical role of the dentist. This book will make an excellent contribution both from the point of view of basic education as well as the continuing education of all dentists and auxiliaries.

Both authors are highly respected and experienced teachers of their subject. They are to be congratulated on producing such a readable and stimulating book on oral medicine. It will undoubtedly contribute to imroved patient care through higher standards of education in this developing field of clinical practice.

D K Mason

Preface

The aim of this book is to provide an outline of the diagnosis and treatment of orofacial conditions which are encompassed in the speciality of oral medicine. As with any evolving clinical field, there will always be advances in the understanding of disease processes, but it is hoped that this text summarizes present-day knowledge and attitudes. It is not feasible to include extensive reference lists in a book of this size, however, a selection of recent original publications, review articles and relevant general texts is included at the end of each chapter to direct the reader to more detailed literature. It is also not possible to provide details of the histopathological features of the conditions described, but such information is readily available in standard texts of oral pathology.

It is hoped that this book will serve as a useful guide, not only for undergraduate or postgraduate dental and medical students but also for the full spectrum of health care workers involved in the management of disease.

M A O Lewis, Cardiff
P-J Lamey, Belfast

Acknowledgements

We are indebted to many of our clinical colleagues who have given us encouragement and support over the years. A special mention must be given to Professor Sir David Mason, Department of Oral Medicine and Pathology, University of Glasgow and Professor Derrick Chisholm, Department of Dental Surgery, University of Dundee, both of whom have been a major source of motivation to us. We are indebted to Professor Roderick Cawson, Emeritus Professor of Oral Medicine and Pathology, University of London, for his constructive criticism of the draft manuscript. We are grateful for the helpful advice given by Professor Robert Johnson, Department of Periodontics, University of Washington, during the preparation of the text. We must thank Mrs Lucy Sayer and Ms Linda Butterworth and Ms Alison Duncan for their continued enthusiasm and advice in helping us throughout this project. Acknowledgement must go to Mrs Linda McGinness and Miss Grace Martin, both of the Department of Oral Medicine and Pathology, University of Glasgow, for typing the original manuscript, and to Mr John Davies and the staff in the Department of Medical Illustration, Glasgow Dental Hospital and School, for producing the illustrations.

Part One
General Background

Chapter 1
The speciality of oral medicine

Dentistry has traditionally been a surgical speciality which has centred around the restoration or extraction of carious teeth, and the provision of dental prostheses. However, improved understanding of disease has revealed the importance of the health of the periodontium and oral mucosa. In addition it is becoming increasingly apparent that changes in the orofacial tissues may be a result of underlying systemic disease. Oral medicine has been defined in a number of ways, but at the present time no one definition has become internationally accepted. At the 1988 World Workshop on Oral Medicine held in Chicago, USA, the following definition was proposed:

Oral Medicine is that area of special competence concerned with the health of and with diseases involving the oral and paraoral structures. It includes those principles of medicine that relate to the mouth, as well as research in biological, pathological, and clinical spheres. Oral medicine includes the diagnosis and medical management of diseases specific to the orofacial tissues and of oral manifestations of systemic diseases. It further includes the management of behavioural disorders and the oral and dental treatment of medically compromised patients.

During the past 25 years there have been significant developments in the field of oral medicine within the UK. Dental schools of several universities now have Chairs of Oral Medicine with active academic departments involved in research and granting of higher degrees. The British Society of Oral Medicine was formed and has advanced the speciality in many ways, especially in providing guidance during the establishment of recognized training programmes in academic oral medicine and the awarding of certificates of accreditation by the Royal Colleges.

Although individuals working in oral medicine ultimately develop particular areas of special expertise and interest, there is a need for such specialists to have a certain level of competence in all aspects of the speciality. Since many oral diseases have a systemic basis there is a clear need to understand how oral medicine relates to other dental and medical specialities. In essence the oral medicine specialist is an oral physician and this is reflected by the structuring of training programmes to involve experience in a variety of clinical areas outside dentistry, such as dermatology, oncology, psychiatry, microbiology, gastroenterology, and radiology.

Further reading

Millard, M. D. and Mason, D. K. (eds) (1988) *Perspectives on 1988 World Workshop on Oral Medicine*, Year Book Medical Publishers, London, pp. v–vi

Chapter 2
Philosophy of care

The taking of the Hippocratic oath confers a responsibility for patient care and assumes that the quality of this care should be of the highest standard. Unfortunately, undergraduate students often fail to appreciate that the clinical teaching being offered to them is primarily directed at improving their diagnostic and management skills. Examinations are a necessary evil; however it is essential that this aspect of their curriculum is not regarded as a means to an end, but is seen to be an exercise that will ultimately help them in the treatment of their patients. Emphasis in this respect should not really be necessary because a conscientious and caring approach to a patient should be an inherent reason why dentistry was initially chosen as a career. Following graduation, all clinicians should undertake further study by: regular reading of professional journals; attendance at postgraduate courses; and the seeking of higher qualifications. Knowledge acquired during such activity can then be used to complement the experience gained during everyday work.

Acceptance of an individual for care assumes the duty not to abandon the patient subsequently if a diagnosis and successful treatment are not achieved. A clinician can interpret this by asking the two questions: 'Have all the appropriate investigations been undertaken?' and 'Is the patient's condition improving?' If the answer to either of these questions is 'No', then it is sensible to seek further professional advice.

Although the vast majority of patients do not expect an individual clinician to be able to deal with every problem, they do expect referral to specialists when appropriate. Failure to provide an adequate service can cause some patients to become critical and lose confidence in their general practitioner or specialist. It is essential, therefore, for the general dental practitioner, general medical practitioner and hospital specialist to be partners in the provision of health care for patients with orofacial problems. Good communication, either by telephone or, preferably, by letter, should be maintained among all clinicians involved in the patient's management. Although attendance at multiple clinics is not ideal, certain patients do require treatment by specialists from various disciplines.

The philosophy of care is a concept which is particularly relevant to oral medicine because patients often have orofacial signs or symptoms that are components of an underlying systemic disease. Few conditions encountered in oral medicine should be considered untreatable, although the efficacy of treatment can vary with a particular disorder or stage of disease. Establishing a team approach among family practitioners and hospital specialists gives the greatest likelihood of providing the patient with successful health care.

Part Two
Principles of Diagnosis

Chapter 3
The clinical interview

Patients expect courtesy and are appreciative of a clinician who listens to their problems. Some consideration should be given to the layout of the surgery so that patients are not distanced by an expanse of desks or equipment. Body language is also important, and in this respect fairly close contact, about 1 m apart, is suitable, with the patient on at least the same eye level as the clinician. Except for children or mentally or physically handicapped people, there is little reason why apparently fit patients should be accompanied into the surgery. Exceptions also include deaf patients who require a companion to communicate via sign language, or patients with a language barrier who need a translator.

It is advisable for medicolegal reasons that a third person, such as a dental surgery assistant, is present during any interview or treatment.

3.1 Clinical history

There is no right or wrong way of obtaining a history provided that a comprehensive assessment has been achieved by the end of the interview. Regardless of the method, it is important to allow the patient to relate the history in his or her own words. It may be difficult in a busy clinic to balance the time needed for a patient to give a full history and the need for brevity, but it is essential not to be pushed into a presumptive diagnosis because of shortage of time. Patients who have been seen by a number of other practitioners or specialists previously can pose particular problems because they often insist on providing every detail of previous opinions and explanations of their complaints. It is only experience which will allow the clinician to tailor the questions to suit the patient and thus maximize the time available.

From the time of the opening question the quality and quantity of the patient's reply should be appreciated because this can provide helpful information. Patients with psychological disorders may either avoid eye contact and speak in an almost audible whisper, or fix their gaze on the clinician and relate their tale in a strident tone. In addition, a patient may exhibit signs of stress, such as clenching the arm-rest of the dental chair firmly, fidgeting with clothing or wringing their hands. Monotonous or repetitive speech is also suggestive of low mood or hypothyroidism. In contrast to this, the use of florid terms in the description of the complaint may indicate the presence of a psychological overlay.

Some patients may appear to have what can best be described as 'evasive finesse': just at the point when the crux of the problem appears to be elucidated the patient will switch the conversation to some trivial side issue. In this circumstance there are basically two possibilities; either the patient is genuinely not aware that he or she is not talking about the problem or the patient is deliberately not providing the clinician with an answer to the questions posed. There are also individuals who almost challenge the clinician to cure them, and this challenge can be perpetuated if the patient fails to give a straightforward reply. This may be due to the fact that the patient has a vested interest in not being cured because they may be receiving invalidity benefits or be undergoing assessment for criminal or industrial injury payments.

Sometimes a patient may adopt the stance of 'I've seen a number of clinicians, so why should you be any better', due to a perceived dislike for health professionals. Alternatively, the patient may blame dentistry for his or her loss of teeth or changed appearance. In these circumstances the patient can become obsessional and it is not surprising that such an individual may have undergone a number of unsuccessful courses of dental treatment in a short period of time. On other occasions marital disharmony may be attributed by one partner as being the result of dental treatment, claiming that the patient's appearance has been altered and the marriage rendered unstable.

The presence of a significant psychological problem should be suspected when a patient arrives at the clinic with a detailed written documentation of his or her complaint. Such documentation is often lengthy and it is only as the interview proceeds that the clinician can decide whether it is helpful, or irrelevant histrionics.

It is against this backdrop of patient-clinician interaction that a history needs to be established. With even the most difficult patient, helpful information can be obtained if the clinical environment is convivial and the history is taken in a sympathetic manner. It is not particularly important whether detailed questions are asked about the orofacial complaints prior to questioning about the patient's general medical history. What is important is that in the course of the consultation the clinician is fully aware of the patient's complaint, is informed about his or her medical status, has formulated a differential diagnosis and has considered relevant investigations and treatment in the light of the patient's general health.

The complaint

The style of history taking is an individual process, but it is useful to establish from the outset whether or not the patient has more than one complaint. In the case of multiple complaints the major problem should be dealt with first, followed by any other complaints in descending order of severity.

Very often it is a complaint of pain, swelling or ulceration which will lead to the patient seeking help. However, mucosal abnormalities, especially early stages of carcinoma, can be painless and the patient may be unaware of their presence unless they have been detected during routine clinical examination by the dentist or doctor. In this situation it is clearly difficult to obtain details of how long any such lesion may have been present or if any change has occurred. Nevertheless a number of aspects of history taking are common to these varied clinical presentations and some basic questions should be asked to ascertain the following features of the complaint:

1. site;
2. when first noticed;
3. when present;
4. precipitating factors;
5. relieving factors.

Further questioning will be determined by the type of complaint.

Pain

In the case of pain it is essential to establish its nature, severity and timing. If asked to describe the pain, patients will often use terms such as dull, sharp, throbbing, nagging, shooting or burning. Most patients have little difficulty in choosing one of these terms to describe their pain, a feature which is helpful in achieving a diagnosis. However, severity of pain is a difficult feature to assess because descriptive words can have widely differing interpretation among individuals. Therefore it is helpful to use a chart or scale to record the severity of the pain. One useful rating is to ask the patient to score the pain on a scale of zero to 10, where zero is 'no pain' and 10 is the 'worst pain experienced'. Such a score will give a good indication of severity and is helpful in monitoring the effect of any subsequent treatment. The patient should be asked if the pain is present every day and, if so, how the pain alters from the time of waking in the morning until going to bed at night. Some patients who are involved in shift work need to have such questions rephrased in relation to their own sleep patterns.

Swelling

The presence and severity of any persistent swelling can be judged by the clinician at the time of examination. However, in a number of conditions swelling may be episodic and absent when the patient attends. In these circumstances the patient should be asked to describe the swelling in terms such as the size of a pea, acorn or walnut. It is also helpful to know whether relatives or friends of the patient have commented on the swelling. In the case of episodic swelling the timing and rapidity of its onset should be determined along with duration of symptoms. The awareness by the patient of any discharge should be noted.

Ulceration

When a patient complains of ulceration it is helpful to establish whether it is the first episode of ulceration or if there have been previous occurrences. In the case of recurrent ulcers information should be obtained on the site(s), number, frequency and duration of any previous lesions. The degree of pain associated with any area of ulceration should also be ascertained.

Summary

It is important during history taking to formulate a likely differential diagnosis as the consultation proceeds. As the story unfolds, known aetiological factors of a possible diagnosis have to be constantly borne in mind and appropriate questions asked. Any aspect of the history which is regarded as being significant to the patient's complaint should be legibly documented in the case notes. In regard to the description of mucosal lesions, a number of special terms can be used, as outlined in Table 3.1 and Figure 3.1. There is an obvious legal reason for recording the clinical history in addition to the general consideration of adequate patient care.

Erosion

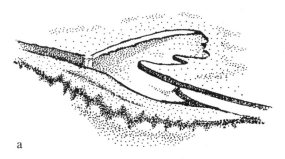

a

Vesicle/Bulla

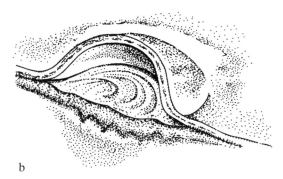

b

Ulcer

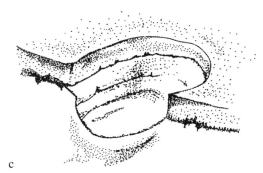

c

Figure 3.1 Diagram of the clinical terms used to describe oral mucosal lesions. (a) Erosion, (b) Vesicle/bulla, (c) Ulcer

Table 3.1 Terminology used to describe oral mucosal lesions

Erosion	A partial loss of the surface epithelium without exposure of the deeper layers or underlying connective tissue
Ulcer	A full thickness loss of the epithelium with exposure of the underlying connective tissue
Vesicle	A small, not more than 5 mm in diameter, circumscribed fluid accumulation. May be intraepithelial and single or multiple
Bulla	A large, greater than 5 mm in diameter, circumscribed fluid accumulation. May be intraepithelial or subepithelial and single or multiple
Plaque	A large circumscribed elevated area
Papule	A small circumscribed elevated area. (This term usually used to describe cutaneous abnormalities rather than mucosal lesions)
Macule	A circumscribed area of discolouration. May be small or large and single or multiple

3.2 Medical history

It is good practice to obtain a signed record of the medical history for each patient who undergoes dental treatment. Medical history forms are commercially available and are basically standardized, although variations in detail do occur among manufacturers. Alternatively, an individual practice or hospital clinic may prefer to construct its own proforma (Figure 3.2). If a proforma is used then the patient can be asked to complete this before the clinical interview, but it is essential that each section is subsequently checked verbally by the clinician. Regardless of the questions asked, it is important to address each point in a colloquial manner. For example, not all patients will know what a cerebrovascular accident is, but the majority are likely to know what a stroke is.

Two major medical reasons for taking an adequate history are, first, awareness of the

CONFIDENTIAL

TITLE:(MR/MS/MRS/MISS).........................   NAME.................................

DATE OF BIRTH..   MALE/FEMALE...............................

ADDRESS...

TEL NO...OCCUPATION...

EXPECTANT MOTHER   YES/NO

	YES	NO	DETAILS
1. Do you feel generally healthy?			
2. Have you had rheumatic fever?			
3. Have you had hepatitis or jaundice?			
4. Do you have any heart complaints such as heart attack, high blood pressure, angina, heart murmur or a replacement heart valve			
5. Do you suffer from bronchitis, asthma, or other chest conditions?			
6. Do you have arthritis?			
7. a) Are you receiving any tablets, creams, ointments from your doctor.			
b) Are you taking or having you taken steroids in the last two years			
8. Are you allergic to any medicine, food or materials?			
9. Are you epileptic or prone to fainting attacks?			
10. Have you ever bleed excessively following a cut or tooth extraction?			
11. Have you been hospitalised? If "Yes", what for and when?			
12. Has the Blood Transfusion Service ever refused your blood?			
13. Are you attending any other Hospital/Clinics or Specialists?			

Doctor's Name and Address   Dentist's Name and Address

....

....

....

Tel No...   Tel No...

Figure 3.2 Medical history form

presence of systemic disease and second, preparedness for any potential medical emergency which the patient may develop. These factors aside, it is now mandatory to obtain a medical history for medicolegal reasons.

Some medical history forms include a section regarding informed consent, which is an increasingly important factor in patient care.

3.3 Social history

In the context of a relevant social history the patients should be asked about marital status, current and past employment, tobacco habits, alcohol intake, drug abuse and previous treatment for anxiety and depression. Many patients find questions regarding their alcohol intake amusing and are likely to discuss psychological factors such as anxiety and depression more freely if these questions are asked immediately after the subject of alcohol has been raised.

The use of a ten-point scale related to social circumstances is helpful in detecting possible adverse social factors. Patients should be asked to rate their social circumstances in the context of how happy they are at home, how well they get on with neighbours, and whether they have any financial or family problems on a scale of zero to 10, where zero means 'things could not be worse' and 10 means 'things could not be better'. Patients giving scores of less than 10 can then be asked 'What would need to happen to make things 10 out of 10?' Such questioning will often focus on a number of important social factors in the patient's lives which may be significant in terms of their oral complaint and avoids the clinician's exhaustive questioning about factors which may be irrelevant.

3.4 Dental history

The dental history should include details of the pattern of dental attendance, the type and age of any prostheses and when they are worn. Details of any removable or fixed orthodontic appliances should be recorded. It can be helpful to ascertain whether the patient thinks that the onset of his or her oral complaint was related to previous dental treatment. For patients who have dental prostheses, questions should be asked about prosthetic hygiene, including details of any solutions which the protheses may be cleaned with or placed in overnight. It is helpful to know whether a patient is a regular or irregular attender because this provides some perspective on the significance he or she puts on oral health.

3.5 Clinical examination

The clinician will have a good opportunity to observe the patient during the taking of the clinical history. This may reveal obvious abnormalities, such as cranial nerve palsies, facial swelling or cutaneous rashes. It is useful for the clinician to observe the frequency of blinking as an increase from 'normal' may indicate xerophthalmia. If the patient is overtly fearful or exhibits signs of imminent tearfulness, this may indicate a significant psychological disorder. As with history taking, there is no correct method of clinical examination so long as all the tissues are adequately examined. The examination can be divided into extraoral and intraoral assessment.

Extraoral assessment

It is logical to carry out the extraoral examination first and this can begin with palpation of the neck for lymphadenopathy. The procedure should be explained to the patient and performed from behind with the collar of any shirt or blouse the patient may be wearing partially undone. All submental, submandibular, posterior auricular and cervical nodes should be palpated in turn. The cervical vertebrae should be palpated and neck movement assessed in lateral movements and on rotation. The parotid salivary glands should be palpated and any enlargement or tenderness noted. In true parotid enlargement there is an outward deflection of the lower part of the ear lobe, the presence of which is best detected by viewing the patient face on. The mandibular condyles should be palpated and the patient asked to perform a full range of jaw movements including maximum opening and lateral excursions. Any limitation of movement or tenderness should be noted. The temporalis and masseter muscles should be palpated with the patient clenching the jaw, to determine bulk and presence of tenderness. It can be helpful to apply pressure to reported areas of pain, such as the maxillary sinuses or temporal arteries.

Intraoral assessment

The clinician must wear surgical gloves to perform the intraoral examination. If the patient wears dentures these should be removed and examined for features such as obvious wear facets or the presence of debris. It may subsequently be necessary to ask the patient to replace the dentures to assess their relationship to any area of mucosal abnormality.

A systematic intraoral examination should be undertaken to ensure that no areas of the mouth are overlooked. The inner aspect of the lips, the hard and soft palate, buccal mucosae, floor of the mouth and dorsum and the lateral margins of the tongue are examined in turn. The lateral margin of the tongue should be examined with the tip of the tongue held with a gauze swab. A record of the teeth present should be made along with a brief evaluation of the distribution of any caries or restorations and the presence of periodontal disease including tooth mobility. The possible relationship between any area of mucosal abnormality and the teeth must be established.

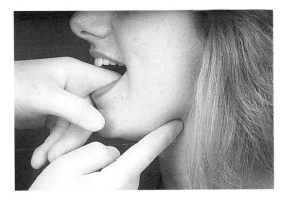

Figure 3.3 Bimanual palpation of the submandibular gland

During examination the amount and consistency of saliva can be determined. As a crude assessment of the saliva, a dental examination mirror should easily lift off the tissues when placed against the buccal mucosae. If xerostomia is present the mirror will stick to the mucosae. The orifices of the parotid and submandibular ducts should be identified. In healthy individuals gentle external palpation of each major salivary gland in turn should give rise to flow of clear saliva from the appropriate duct. Bimanual palpation of the submandibular salivary glands should be undertaken to determine the presence of any enlargement or tenderness (Figure 3.3). Care should be taken to differentiate submandibular gland tenderness from tenderness of the medial pterygoid muscle, or the presence of cervical lymphadenopathy.

Cranial nerves

Examination of the cranial nerves is essential because patients with a neuropathy as part of an underlying illness may initially present in the dental surgery. Nerve function can be assessed relatively easily, although specialized equipment is required to examine fully some cranial nerves such as the optic nerve and the vestibulocochlear nerve.

I The olfactory nerve

The olfactory nerve is responsible for the perception of smell. Impaired function may be detected by asking the patient to identify (with eyes closed) a selection of character-istic substances, such as coffee, orange peel, lemon, soap or peppermint. Substances with strong odours should be avoided because irritation of the nasal mucosa may stimulate the sensory component of the trigeminal nerve and give misleading results. Loss of smell (anosmia) is usually a result of local inflammation such as that due to a common cold rather than a lesion of the nerve itself. Rarer causes of altered sensations of smell include fractures of the ethmoid complex, epilepsy, migraine, phenytoin therapy and psychological disorders.

II Optic nerve

The optic nerve is responsible for the sensa-tion of sight. Drooping of the eyelid (ptosis) or protrusion of the eye with lid retraction (exophthalmos) are possible indications of underlying disease. Unilateral exophthalmos is suggestive of the presence of a tumour of the orbit or thrombosis of the cavernous sinus, whilst bilateral lesions may indicate hyperthyroidism. External examination of the eye may reveal other changes in the conjunctiva and sclera. Subconjunctival haemorrhage is often seen in association with local trauma such as zygomatic arch or nasal fracture. Ulceration of the conjunctiva may occur along with oral ulceration in Behçet's disease. Alterations in the colour of the sclera can be an indication of underlying disease. Blue discoloration has been asso-ciated with osteogenesis imperfecta, whilst a yellow coloration of the sclera is frequently seen in association with the elevated bili-rubin levels which can occur in patients with viral hepatitis. Corneal scarring (pterygium) can occur in (benign) mucous membrane pemphigoid and should be noted.

Integrity of vision may be crudely assessed by perception of light or by asking the patient to count fingers held in front of each eye. Because disease affecting the visual pathway may produce restricted acuity in different areas, the fingers should be held in the central part of the field of vision. This type of test simply reveals whether or not sight is present. A more accurate evaluation is made using Snellen's type charts placed at a distance of 6 m from the patient.

Visual fields may be assessed conveniently in the surgery by the confrontation test. This compares the clinician's field of vision with that of the patient. Seated approximately 1 m away from the clinician, and at the same height, the patient is asked to cover his or her left eye and look directly with the right eye at the clinician's left eye. The clinician covers his or her right eye and places his or her left hand outside the periphery of the field of vision at a point equidistant from him or her and the patient. The finger is then gradually brought into the field of vision and the patient is asked to indicate when it becomes visible. The examiner's awareness of the fingers in the field of vision is used as the control. Each eye is tested independently and in this way the integrity of the nasal, temporal, superior and inferior areas of each eye can be assessed. The location of any pathology is assessed by the extent and pattern of visual field loss (Figure 3.4).

The light reflex is tested by shining a beam of light from an ophthalmoscope into the side of one of the patient's eyes. Care should be taken not to shine the light from directly in front of the eye as this will produce constriction of the pupil due to an accom-modation reaction. In the absence of any nerve dysfunction, a beam of light directed into an eye produces constriction of the pupil not only of that eye (direct reflex) but also of the other eye (consensual reflex). By testing each eye independently it is possible to assess whether a fault is due to failure to detect light in one eye (indicating an optic nerve dysfunction) or failure of pupillary constriction in the other (indicating an auto-nomic dysfunction).

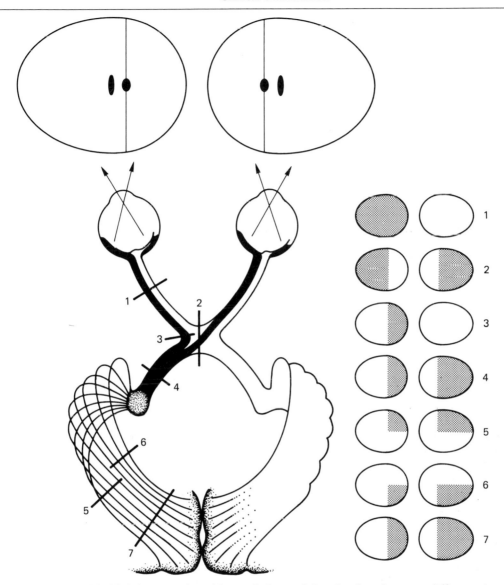

Figure 3.4 Visual field defects produced by pathology of the visual pathway at different sites (1–7) the site of lesion is indicated on the left of the figure and the result and loss of vision of each eye on the right. Shaded areas represent visual loss in the right and/or left eye

III Oculomotor nerve, IV Trochlear nerve and VI Abducens nerve

Three nerves (III, IV and VI) supply extra-ocular muscles which control movement of the eye. The oculomotor nerve (III) supplies all the extrinsic muscles of the eye, apart from the superior oblique which is supplied by the trochlear nerve (IV) and lateral rectus which is supplied by the abducens nerve (V). In addition, the oculomotor nerve contains motor fibres to levator palpebrae superioris producing elevation of the upper eyelid and parasympathetic fibres to sphincter pupillae muscles responsible for constriction of the pupil. Disorders of ocular movement are assessed by asking the patient to follow a point, usually the tip of the examiner's finger, in vertical, horizontal and diagonal directions. To maintain binocular vision, the tip of the examiner's finger should be held not less than 50 cm from the patient.

Complete loss of function of the III, IV or VI cranial nerve, will result in the following clinical signs;

III oculomotor nerve – ptosis with dilated and non-reactive pupil; the eye will be abducted and looking down;
IV trochlear nerve – inability to look downwards and inwards;
VI abducens nerve – diplopia and inability to look laterally.

V Trigeminal nerve

The trigeminal nerve has three main divisions, ophthalmic, maxillary and mandibular, all of which contain sensory fibres that supply the majority of the tissues of the orofacial region including the sinuses and conjunctiva. The mandibular division also contains motor fibres to the muscles of mastication. Sensory function should be assessed by touching the affected area lightly with a material such as a wisp of cotton wool. Assessment is based on a comparison of the right and left sides of the face. If loss of sensation is detected by the soft touch method then it should be confirmed by the use of light touch with a sharp object such as a pin or dental probe.

Motor function can be assessed by asking the patient to open his or her mouth and perform lateral mandibular movements. The extent of movement should be noted and the power can be gauged by providing manual resistance to these movements.

Two reflexes, the corneal reflex and jaw jerk, may be demonstrated when assessing the trigeminal nerve. The corneal reflex is demonstrated by touching the cornea of one eye with a wisp of cotton wool whilst the patient looks to one side. This should lead to blinking of both eyes. In the jaw jerk, tapping

a forefinger which is held on the patient's chin below the lip should result in reflex closure of the mouth.

VII Facial nerve

The facial nerve provides motor innervation to the muscles of facial expression and stapedius muscle. It also travels in close proximity to the nervus intermedius which contains sensory fibres of taste (via the chorda tympani) from the anterior two-thirds of the tongue. The function of the facial nerve can be assessed by asking the patient to smile, whistle or close his or her eyes tightly. Reduced nerve function manifests as drooping of the corner of the mouth, and the inability to frown, smile, whistle or completely close the eyes (Figure 3.5). The

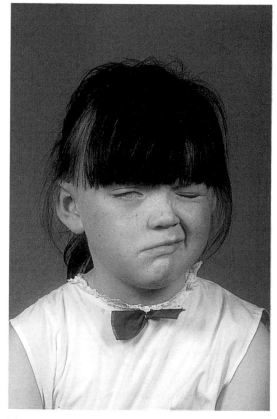

Figure 3.5 Facial nerve palsy

patient should be asked to raise his or her eyebrows, and this will not be possible on the affected side if a lower motor neurone lesion is present, but may be unaffected in upper motor neurone lesions. Causes of upper motor neurone lesions include cerebrovascular accidents, tumours and demyelinating disease. An acute onset of a lower motor neurone defect is often referred to as Bell's palsy. Gradual loss of motor function over a period of time is suggestive of the presence of a tumour of the cerebellopontine angle or parotid gland.

Testing of taste

Taste perception is still a grey scientific area. It is, however, claimed that the four primary tastes (sweet, salt, sour and bitter) can be tested by placing appropriate substances on the surface of the tongue. Solutions of sugar, salt, vinegar and quinine can be applied to the lateral margins of the tongue whilst the tip is held gently with a gauze swab. Patients should perform a mouth rinse with water between substances. Passage of electric currents through the tongue (electrogustometry) will cause a metallic taste. This phenomenon is used in an electronic gustometer which produces a variable passage of current. Patients with intact taste function should have a threshold of approximately 20 µA.

VIII Vestibulocochlear nerve

The vestibulocochlear nerve is made up of two parts, the cochlear nerve which is responsible for hearing and the vestibular nerve which provides information concerning balance. The cochlear nerve may be tested crudely by asking the patient to repeat words or numbers whispered into the ear whilst the other ear is covered.

Rinne's test involves a vibrating (256 Hz or 512 Hz) tuning fork placed over the mastoid bone and the patient is asked to indicate when the sound fades and is no longer heard. The fork is then removed from the mastoid and the vibrating end held close to,

but not touching, the external ear: in health the patient should be able to hear the sound once again.

In Weber's test, the tuning fork is placed on the forehead or vertex and the patient is asked to indicate whether there is a difference in intensity of sound from one side to the other. In health the sound should appear to be in the mid-line with no preference to either side. In perceptive deafness the sound is heard less well on the affected side. In conductive deafness the sound is heard better in the affected side. Definitive testing of the nerve requires audiometry.

IX Glossopharyngeal nerve

The glossopharyngeal nerve is sensory to the posterior third of the tongue (including taste), pharynx, middle ear and Eustachian tube. It carries motor fibres to the stylopharyngeus muscle and an autonomic component (parasympathetic) to the parotid gland.

Testing of the glossopharyngeal nerve is based on the gag reflex which also involves fibres from the vagus nerve. If the pharynx is touched with a spatula then stimulation of the sensory (afferent) fibres of the glossopharyngeal nerve should produce motor (efferent) activity in the vagus nerve which will result in bilateral elevation of the soft palate.

X Vagus nerve

The vagus nerve provides motor supply to the palate, larynx and pharynx. In addition, the vagus contains sensory fibres which carry visceral sensation, and autonomic fibres which supply the heart, bronchi and gastrointestinal tract. The function of the oropharyngeal component of the vagus nerve is assessed by asking the patient to open the mouth and say 'Ah', which involves a bilateral and equal rise of the soft palate. In a unilateral lesion the palate is drawn to the healthy side. If a patient complains of hoarseness of the voice, then the vocal cords should be examined by direct laryngoscopy.

PATIENTS REFERRAL LETTER

DENTAL HOSPITAL
HEATH PARK
CARDIFF CF4 4XY

Tel. No.

Please give my patient an appointment to attend the Department specified below:-

Exam & Emergency	Oral Medicine	
Childrens Dentistry	Orthodontics	
Conservation	Periodontology	
Oral Surgery	Prosthetics	
	T.M.J.	

I wish the patient to be seen by .... if possible

(If a specific Consultant is not nominated, the patient will be given the earliest possible appointment in the speciality)

G.P. Stamp

FOR HOSPITAL USE ONLY

CONSULTANT

DATE: /   /   at

Surname or Family Name:

Date of Birth:

First Names:

Occupation:

Address:

Post Code

Telephone No.:

Male

Female

FOI   NHS Number:

This referral is

| URGENT | |
| NOT URGENT | |

For

Opinion Only	
Diagnosis & Planning	
Emergency Treatment	
Complete Treatment	

LETTER

Dear

.... 19 ....

Re .... Age ....

G.P.'s Signature ....

Please indicate details of DRUG therapy and SENSITIVITY

Figure 3.6 Example of a standard referral letter

XI Spinal accessory nerve

The spinal accessory nerve supplies motor fibres to the sternomastoid and trapezius muscles. To test function the patient is asked to turn the head to one side whilst resistance is provided to the movement by the investigator holding a hand against the jaw. During this procedure the contralateral sternomastoid muscle should contract and become apparent clinically. The bulk and consistency of the muscle can be assessed by palpation. Integrity of the nerve supply to the trapezius is assessed by asking the patient to shrug the shoulders against the resistance of the investigator's hands.

XII Hypoglossal nerve

The hypoglossal nerve supplies motor fibres to the intrinsic and extrinsic muscles of the tongue other than palatoglossus. Hypoglossal function is tested by asking the patient to protrude the tongue. In a unilateral lesion the tongue will deviate to the affected side. The power of the tongue can be assessed by asking the patient to push the tongue into the buccal mucosa whilst the examiner holds a finger on the overlying cheek.

3.6 Referral for a specialist opinion

If a patient requires referral for a specialist opinion then this should be made by letter, although in the case of an emergency an appointment time or advice may be obtained by telephone. Direct verbal communication between the general practitioner and the specialist can be used to gain advice concerning possible drug interactions in relation to oral disease or to provide additional confidential information about a patient which was not included in the referral letter.

The style of the referral letters received in specialist units tends to fall into two categories; the 'please see and treat' type, with virtually no clinical information; or the full letter, which includes details of the complaint along with a provisional diagnosis. Regional hospitals and specialist services often have their own standard referral letter (Figure 3.6), and whenever possible this type of form should be used. If a standard letter is not available then the referral letter should be written in such a way that it includes the following information:

1. Name, address and telephone number of the referring practitioner.
2. Name, address, age and sex of the patient.
3. Reason for referral, including case history, clinical signs and symptoms and provisional diagnosis.
4. Information on relevant medical history and recent treatment, especially drug therapy.
5. Results of recent special investigations, particularly any radiographs (to avoid unnecessary repeated exposure to radiation) should be enclosed.
6. Indication whether an opinion and/or treatment is requested.

Further reading

Scully, C. (1988) The history, diagnosis and treatment planning. In *Clinical Dentistry in Health and Disease, Vol. I The Dental Patient* (ed. C. Scully), Butterworth-Heinemann, Oxford, pp. 7–61

Chapter 4
Special investigations

Special investigations are an everyday aspect of the practice of oral medicine. However, there is no place for the undertaking of repeated investigations, and the appropriateness of any test should be considered carefully. In an increasingly financially aware society it would rightly be considered a waste of resources to screen patients for numerous diseases, although additional investigations will often be undertaken in hospital for research or epidemiological purposes. Ethical approval and patient permission should always be sought before carrying out any test which could be regarded as additional to those necessary for patient care.

The recent trend of dental and medical practitioners working together in Health Centres or Primary Care Units has made it easier to perform the range of special investigations which an individual patient may require, because the necessary equipment and means of transporting specimens to the laboratory are freely available. In general practice, obtaining and forwarding samples to the laboratory may be difficult. In this situation the dentist should either obtain necessary equipment and arrange transport of the samples him or herself or should request that the tests are performed by the patient's general medical practitioner or local specialist clinic. The practice of dentistry is changing and there is increasing scope for the dental practitioner to undertake basic special investigations. A major advantage of performing initial tests within the practice is that it improves dentist-patient contact and enhances the role of the dental practitioner in overall patient health care. In addition it is often easier for patients to attend their local practice rather than the district clinic or hospital. Advice and necessary equipment for haematological, microbiological and histopathological investigations can be obtained from the local health centre or hospital. Special regulations apply where it is necessary to send clinical samples by post. Specimens for pathological or microbiological investigation need to be clearly marked 'pathology specimen' and sent in a bag which will absorb fixation or culture fluid in the event of damage. It is the clinician's responsibility to ensure that any specimen is correctly packaged and labelled. The accompanying request form must be completed in full, since the laboratory may refuse to process the specimen if inadequate details have been provided.

4.1 Interpreting the laboratory report

The interpretation of laboratory data clearly depends on an understanding of what is normal for the age and sex of the patient. The laboratory to which samples are sent should provide a reference list of normal values because results can vary widely depending on the assay method used and the format in which they are expressed. The normal range of values for a particular test is usually calculated from a statistical evaluation of values obtained from a healthy population. Assuming that the values will be normally distributed around a mean, then by definition 95% of individuals will have a value which is within plus or minus two standard deviations from the mean.

Whenever an abnormality is found the clinician should ask the question 'How reliable is the test?' Fortunately the vast majority of laboratory tests are accurate and appropriate action can be taken on the result(s) obtained. However, assessment of certain factors, such as levels of vitamin B_{12} or folic acid, can be unreliable and if a marginally abnormal result is obtained then it is often worthwhile repeating the test in the first instance.

4.2 Emergency laboratory investigations

For the majority of conditions, it is not necessary to obtain the results of an investigation immediately. However, laboratory results are required as a matter of urgency for patients who are suspected of having certain serious underlying diseases. In these circumstances the sample should be transported to the laboratory immediately and the laboratory contacted by telephone to inform them of the urgency of the specimen. Clinical conditions which may present in the dental surgery and require urgent investigation include the blood dyscrasias: leukaemia, thrombocytopenia, agranulocytosis and aplastic anaemia. If any of these conditions is suspected then a full blood count and film must be performed. The half life of platelets is short (10 days) and therefore thrombocytopenia (platelet count less than $150 \times 10^9/l$) is regarded as a medical emergency which requires immediate hospitalization for transfusion to avoid intracranial bleeding.

Giant cell arteritis, an uncommon but important cause of facial pain, also represents an emergency since there is a risk of irreversible blindness. It tends to affect the elderly, and can be diagnosed when the erythrocyte sedimentation rate (ESR) is greatly raised (over 100 mm/h).

The patient's general medical practitioner should be informed immediately of any abnormal laboratory findings.

4.3 Assessment of HIV status

Establishment of a positive human immuno-deficiency virus status has far-reaching implications, and therefore investigation of potential HIV infection should never be undertaken without prior professional counselling of the patient. Appropriate counselling can be arranged via the patient's general medical practitioner, local genitourinary clinic or regional infectious disease unit.

4.4 Venepuncture

The antecubital fossa is the site of choice for venepuncture because the veins are larger than those on the dorsum of the hand which may be used occasionally but are technically difficult to enter and readily collapse. Once the necessary equipment (Table 4.1) is assembled the procedure of venepuncture should be explained to the patient. A tourniquet, which is available in small, medium and large sizes, should be applied midway between the elbow and shoulder. At this time patients often start to contract the muscles of their arm to make veins more prominent, but this is not necessary.

A large vein, which is usually detectable by visual inspection or palpation, is then sought in the antecubital fossa, taking care to avoid superficial veins because they are too small to permit adequate sampling (Figure 4.1). The plunger of the syringe should be depressed fully before use, otherwise it can stick as a consequence of the manufacturing

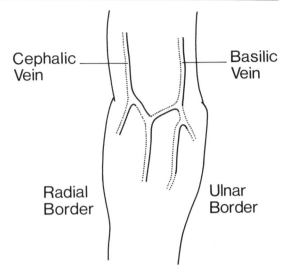

Figure 4.1 Veins of the right arm

sterilization procedure. A needle or butterfly which are both colour-coded as blue (23 gauge), green (21 gauge) or white (19 gauge) should be attached to the syringe. Generally a 21 gauge size is chosen because the narrow bore of the 23 gauge results in a slow blood flow, which is a disadvantage if more than 10 ml has to be obtained. Insertion of a gauge 19 needle is painful and the bore is unnecessarily large for routine purposes.

Venepuncture, can be complicated by fear of the procedure, particularly in children. For such patients it is as well to have all equipment ready before the child enters the surgery. A parent may wish to hold the child's arm if it reassures the child and does not unduly delay the procedure. The parent should be discouraged from making comments such as 'This will not hurt' and 'Be brave' as such statements usually heighten the child's anxiety. The procedure outlined in Table 4.2 should be followed.

4.5 Haematological investigations

A variety of tests based on the examination of the patient's blood are useful in the

Table 4.1 Equipment for venepuncture

Tourniquet
Cleansing (alcohol) swab
Needle or butterfly (19 or 21 gauge for adults, 21 or 23 gauge for children)
Syringe (5, 10, 20 or 50 ml)
Gauze swab
Sample containers
Sticking plaster
Micropore tape

Table 4.2 Procedure for venepuncture in antecubital fossa

1. Apply tourniquet to upper arm
2. Identify vein, usually by palpation
3. Prepare overlying skin with swab
4. Insert needle with the bevel uppermost at 45° angle to skin (blood will appear at base of needle when the vein is entered)
5. Withdraw desired amount of blood slowly (avoid rapid removal because it may cause haemolysis of red cells)
6. Release tourniquet
7. Place gauze swab over puncture site prior to removal of needle
8. Remove needle from syringe and dispose in a box for 'sharps'
9. Fill bottles to appropriate levels and cap. Gently invert or roll tubes containing anticoagulants
10. Dispose of syringe in a box for 'sharps'
11. Check venepuncture site has stopped bleeding and apply sticking plaster (use gauze swab under micropore tape if the patient has a hypersensitivity to sticking plaster)
12. Label bottles and package with appropriate forms

diagnosis of orofacial disease. The number of tests and techniques now available is large, but the samples required for those haematological and biochemical investigations which are used most frequently in oral medicine are outlined in Table 4.3.

Full blood count

A full blood count provides the following information; total and differential white blood cell count (WBC), red blood cell count (RBC), haemoglobin (Hb), haematocrit (HCT), mean corpuscular volume (MCV), mean corpuscular haemoglobin (MCH) and platelet count (PLAT). Changes in any of these variables can indicate the presence of underlying disease (Table 4.4).

Blood film

Examination of the blood film will detect abnormalities in shape and staining of the red cells. In addition, the relative proportions of various white cells (differential count) can be obtained. In health the leukocytes consist of a mixture of lymphocytes, monocytes, polymorphonuclear neutrophils, eosinophils and basophils. The appearance of myelocytes, myeloblasts and lymphoblasts in the blood would be an indication of the presence of leukaemia.

Iron

Assessment of iron status can be performed in two ways: either the ratio of serum iron (Fe) to total iron binding capacity (TIBC) in which a value of less than 16% saturation is considered to indicate iron deficiency, or measurement of ferritin, with a level below 25 ng/ml indicating deficiency.

Established iron deficiency will result in a microcytosis and reduced haemoglobin (iron deficiency anaemia). The detection of iron deficiency accompanied by a normal haemoglobin is termed sideropenia (latent iron deficiency).

Vitamin B_{12}

Vitamin B_{12} is involved in erythrocyte production and deficiency of vitamin B_{12} should be suspected if a macrocytosis is detected in a full blood count and film.

Vitamin B_{12} is estimated by a radioimmunoassay of serum. The assay is sometimes unreliable and it is worthwhile repeating the test if a low B_{12} value is obtained in conjunction with a normal MCV.

Folic acid

Folic acid is involved in erythrocyte production, and deficiency of folic acid should be suspected if a macrocytosis is detected in a full blood count and film. Apart from deficiencies due to anticonvulsant drug therapy and increased demand in pregnancy, the cause of low levels of folate are alcoholism

Table 4.3 Haematological and biochemical investigations

Test	Sample	Comment
Haematology		
Full blood count	Pink top EDTA bottle 5 ml	Invert bottle 2–3 times after filling
Corrected whole blood folate	Pink top EDTA bottle 5 ml	Invert bottle 2–3 times after filling
Vitamin B_{12}	White top plain tube 10 ml	
Ferritin	Pink top EDTA 5 ml	Preferable to serum iron and total iron binding capacity
Erythrocyte sedimentation rate	Purple Westergren bottle	Send to laboratory immediately
Clotting screen	Variable	Check with laboratory
Biochemistry		
Glucose		
(a) Random	Yellow top fluoride bottle 2–5 ml	Patient fasted overnight prior to collection
(b) Tolerance test	Yellow top fluoride bottle 2–5 ml	Two samples: Initial fasted then second sample 2 hours after oral administration of 75 g glucose
Alkaline phosphatase Gammaglutamyl transpeptidase (gamma GT) Alanine transaminase (ALT) Asparate transaminase (AST)	White top plain tube 10 ml	
Sodium Potasium Urea Calcium Phosphate Total protein Albumin	White top plain tube 10 ml	Calcium levels should be acquired with tourniquet off
Cortisol		
(a) Random	White top plain 10 ml	Collect at 08.00–09.00 h
(b) Synacthen test	White top plain 10 ml	Two samples; initial sample as random 08.00–09.00 hours. Second sample 30 minutes after i.v. or i.m. administration of 0.25 mg tetracosactrin (Synacthen)
Growth hormone	White top plain 10 ml	Send samples along with glucose tolerance test
Tri-iodothyroinine (T3) Thyroxine (T4) Free thyroxine index (FTI)	White top plain 20 ml	Plastic or glass container — check with laboratory

and malabsorption due to diseases such as coeliac disease. Estimations of serum folate are of little use and determination of corrected whole blood folate is the appropriate test.

Erythrocyte sedimentation rate (ESR)

If anticoagulated blood (oxalated, citrated or heparinized) from a healthy adult is left to

Table 4.4 Interpretation of haematological results

Test	Level raised	Level reduced
White cell count (WBC)	Pregnancy; infection; leukaemia	Early leukaemia; drug reaction; idiopathic; some infections; bone marrow disease
Differential WBC		
Neutrophils	Pregnancy; infection; leukaemia; malignancy	Drug reaction; idiopathic; some infections; bone marrow disease
Lymphocytes	Some infections; leukaemia; bowel disease	Some infections; AIDS
Eosinophils	Atopy; some infections; lymphoma	Some immune disorders
Red cell count (RBC)	Polycythaemia	Anaemia
Haemoglobin (Hb)	Polycythaemia; myeloproliferative disorders	Anaemia
Haematocrit (HCT)	Polycythaemia	Anaemia
Mean cell volume (MCV)	Vitamin B_{12} deficiency; folate deficiency; alcoholism; liver disease	Iron deficiency; thalassaemia
Mean cell haemoglobin (MCH)	Pernicious anaemia	Iron deficiency; thalassaemia
Platelets (PLAT)	Myeloproliferative disorders	Drug reaction; leukaemia; infections; idiopathic

stand the erythrocytes sediment at a rate of approximately 15 mm in 1 hour. However, in a number of conditions, in particular chronic inflammatory disease, malignancy, or acute infection, the sedimentation rate is greatly increased. The processes involved in this phenomenon are not fully understood, but it is likely to involve changes in levels of plasma proteins. The ESR is routinely assessed using the Westergren method.

Clotting screen

A history of prolonged bleeding may represent a reduced level or function of the platelets, low levels of clotting factors or anticoagulant therapy. If a bleeding disorder is suspected a full blood count and measurements of prothrombin time (PT) and activated partial thromboplastin time (APTT) should be performed. Levels of specific clotting factors can also be measured.

Sickle cell disorders

The Sickledex test is used to detect an abnormal form of haemoglobin, haemoglobin S, which occurs in sickle cell trait and sickle cell disease. These conditions are inherited and occur most frequently in individuals of African, Mediterranean or Middle Eastern origin.

4.6 Biochemical investigations

Venous plasma blood glucose

Estimation of blood glucose level should be made first thing in the morning after an overnight fast. If a raised random venous plasma blood glucose level is detected a glucose tolerance test (GTT) should be performed. The GTT consists of taking an initial blood sample and a further sample 2 hours later following a 75 g glucose drink.

Table 4.5 Interpretation of biochemical values

Factor	Level reduced	Level raised
Sodium	Addison's disease; renal failure	Cushing's disease, dehydration
Potassium	Diabetes, therapeutic use of diuretics, Cushing's disease	Addison's disease, renal failure
Urea	Liver disease; nephrotic syndrome	Renal failure, dehydration
Calcium	Hypoparathyroidsm; renal failure	Hyperparathyroidism
Phosphate	Hyperparathyroidism; renal failure	Hypoparathyroidism; hypervitaminosis D
Total protein	Renal failure; myelomatosis	Liver disease
Albumin	Liver disease; malabsorption	Dehydration
Alkaline phosphatase	Hypothyroidsm	Paget's disease; fibrous dysplasia; bone malignancy; liver disease; hyperparathyroidism
Gamma GT		Liver disease
ALT		Liver disease; infectious mononucleosis
AST		Liver disease
Uric acid	Liver disease	Leukaemia; renal failure; myelomatosis; alcohol abuse

Profile

A biochemical profile, performed on a clotted 10 ml sample of venous blood, will provide a range of information that is useful in diagnosis (Table 4.5).

Cortisol

Measurement of cortisol levels is useful in the detection of Addison's disease or adrenal suppression following corticosteroid therapy. Adrenal response is assessed by monitoring levels of cortisol before and 30 minutes after intravenous or intramuscular administration of 0.25 mg tetracosactrin, a synthetic analogue of ACTH (Synacthen test).

Growth hormone

Assessment of levels of growth hormone is required in the diagnosis of gigantism and acromegaly. This should be done along with a glucose tolerance test.

Thyroid function test

Thyroid function tests may give conflicting results, and no single test is sufficiently reliable or informative. Measurement should therefore involve assays of tri-iodothyronine (T3), thyroxine (T4) and free thyroxine index.

4.7 Immunological investigations

Full blood count

It could be argued that the white blood cell count (with differential subpopulations if required) of a full blood count is a basic assessment of immunological status. Such an investigation can indicate whether a patient has a mild reduction in white cell numbers or a profound reduction in the white cell series (neutropenia). It will also reveal if white blood cell numbers are extremely high, as in leukaemia.

A laboratory technique known as fluorescent automated cell sorter analysis (FACS) is now able to determine individual lymphocyte subpopulations, particularly numbers of T-helper (CD4) cells and T-suppressor (CD8) cells. Such analysis has become important because a decline in CD4 cells and the CD4:CD8 ratio is characteristic of the immune deficit seen in patients with HIV infection and AIDS.

Immunoglobulins

A variety of techniques, including radioimmunoassay (RIA), radioallergo-sorbent-testing (RAST) and enzyme-linked immunoassay (ELISA) are available to quantify immunoglobulin levels. Immunoglobulin electrophoresis can separate individual immunoglobulins and, by co-chromatography with antibody to kappa and lambda light chains, determine whether a given increase in immunoglobulin levels is polyclonal or monoclonal. In a polyclonal gammopathy the increased immunoglobulins present have equal numbers of either kappa or lambda chains, whereas in a monoclonal gammopathy one light chain type predominates.

Multiple myeloma and Waldenström's macroglobulinaemia can both present in the oral cavity and are examples of conditions in which immunological studies are invaluable in diagnosis.

Autoantibodies

Determination of the presence and titres of autoantibodies is useful in the diagnosis of connective tissue disease, bullous disorders and pernicious anaemia.

Antinuclear factor and rheumatoid factor

Antinuclear factor (ANF) is detected by means of immunofluorescence. The patient's sera is placed onto sections of rat liver and both the staining pattern and the highest dilution (titre) at which staining is achieved are estimated. ANF is detectable in the serum of patients with systemic lupus erythematosis (SLE) and in some cases of discoid lupus erythematosis (DLE). If a high ANF titre is present the serum is also tested for antibodies for both single-stranded and double-stranded DNA. Many drugs can produce lupus-like syndromes and demonstrate high ANF titres, but antibodies to single-stranded DNA should not be present.

Rheumatoid factor, which is an immunoglobulin against the patient's own immunoglobulins, is usually measured by radioimmunoassay and is a common feature of rheumatoid arthritis. Not all patients with rheumatoid arthritis have rheumatoid factor and those who do not are termed sero-negative. Connective tissue diseases are important because they can involve the oral cavity and associated structures, including the mandible, temporomandibular joint, teeth and salivary glands.

Antibodies to stratified squamous epithelium

Indirect immunofluorescence can be used to detect the presence of autoantibodies to stratified squamous epithelium which occur in pemphigus and pemphigoid.

Parietal cell antibody and intrinsic factor antibody

Antibodies to gastric parietal cells and intrinsic factor are detectable in the serum of patients with pernicious anaemia.

Complement

Complement consists of a complex of serum enzymatic proteins which is activated by the alternative and classical pathways. Individual components can be measured in addition to overall integrity of the system. Hereditary angioedema is characterized by a reduced level of C-I esterase inhibitor and detection of this is diagnostic.

There is increasing interest in functional immunological investigations which are clinically useful when polymorphonuclear leucocyte numbers are present in normal numbers but have abnormal function. Decreased immunological activity is present in Chediak-Higashi syndrome or Di-George's syndrome, the latter being an example of isolated T-cell deficiency.

Human lymphocyte antigen

At present, assessment of human lymphocyte antigen (HLA) status is usually limited to specialist laboratories for research purposes. An individual's genetic make-up is an important factor in susceptibility to a variety of systemic conditions, including those which produce oral diseases. HLA typing is useful in the diagnosis of Behçet's disease and Reiter's syndrome.

4.8 Urinalysis

The composition of urine is complex but analysis is often useful in detection of disease. Determination of the levels of glucose, blood, protein, ketones, bilirubin or urobilinogen in the urine can often indicate the presence of disease. A number of commercial systems which give a rapid measurement of urinary constituents are available for use at the bedside or in the surgery. They should only be regarded as rough indicators, and if an abnormality is detected more definitive investigation is indicated. A midstream specimen of urine (MSSU) is collected to avoid variations which occur at the beginning and end of micturition.

4.9 Microbiological Investigations

Viral infection

Although it is now possible to identify a number of viruses by isolation techniques, this technique is only often used for *Herpes*

simplex virus. In primary herpetic gingivostomatitis a swab of an ulcerated lesion is placed in virus transport medium, a salt solution which contains antibiotics and antifungal agents to limit the growth of bacteria and fungi. In the laboratory an aliquot of the sample is inoculated on a prepared confluent layer of baby hamster kidney (BHK) cells in tissue culture. The culture is incubated for approximately 10 days at 37°C, at which time the virus can be identified by immunofluorescence methods. Identical isolation regimes can be employed in other *Herpes simplex* virus infections, such as herpes labialis or recurrent intraoral herpetic infections.

Serological evidence of viral infection is particularly useful when the patient is exposed to a virus for the first time. In primary herpetic gingivostomatitis, a blood sample taken early in the disease (acute phase sera) and a sample taken 14 days later (convalescent sera) will contain different amounts of immunoglobulin directed towards the virus. A complement fixation test enables quantification of the amount of virus-specific immunoglobulin present. The titre of antibody in the convalescent sera should show at least a four-fold rise from that detected in the acute phase sera. The titre is defined as the maximum dilution at which antibody is still detectable; the higher the dilution at which immunoglobulin is still identified, the greater the amount of such immunoglobulin present. Because doubling dilutions of the patient's sera are used in the test, if the initial titre is 1:16 then the convalescent titre has to be at least four dilutions higher, at 1:256, to confirm clinical diagnosis. This same principle can be applied to many viral infections, although some laboratories are limited in the range of tests which are routinely available. In recurrent herpes labialis, there will be no increase in circulating immunoglobulin because the virus travels directly from cell to cell and thus evades the host immune reponse.

The interpretation of virological data should be straightforward: either *Herpes simplex* virus has or has not been successfully isolated or there has or has not been a significant change in antibody titre. Interestingly, response to Herpes simplex virus infection may sometimes involve production of immunoglobulin to the closely related virus Varicella zoster and therefore a false positive may be observed, so-called amnestic response.

Fungal infection

Diagnosis of oral candidosis is usually based on culture of the organism on Sabourand's agar or Pagano-Levin medium. The samples required for investigation of oral candidosis will depend to some extent on the type of candidal infection present. Swabs of lesional sites and the fitting surface of any denture worn are essential. Smears, which can be prepared by scraping the lesion tissue with a flat plastic instrument and spreading the cells on to a glass slide before staining using Gram's method, are also helpful.

Sampling of the oral mucosa for candidal carriage using an oral rinse technique, which involves vigorous rinsing of the mouth with 10 ml of phosphate buffered saline, has the advantage of allowing quantification of the candidal load (Figure 4.2).

It is important to realize that in angular cheilitis the oral cavity is the reservoir of candidal infection and the anterior nares is the reservoir of staphyloccal infection. The clinical appearance of angular cheilitis does not allow the clinician to determine the identity of infecting organisms. However, Gram staining of the smears from each angle of the mouth can rapidly provide information on the likely presence of Candida and/or Staphylococci.

Culture of candidal species will confirm that the yeast is present and allow species identification. Although a variety of candidal species have been isolated from oral lesions, no particular species appears to be more pathogenic than any other. It is now possible to biotype candidal species by means of sugar fermentation tests. This has potential clinical implications, because it will enable evaluation of the role of individual candidal biotypes in a given pathological process. Culture is often combined with sensitivity testing to the antifungal agents nystatin or amphotericin B. *In vitro* resistance to candida can occasionally be seen, but in practice drug resistance is not a clinical problem. An exception to this has been encountered in some HIV positive patients treated with systemic antifungal therapy.

4.10 Histopathological investigations

Biopsy

A biopsy is undertaken to confirm a clinical diagnosis or obtain information which will provide a diagnosis. The patient's medical history should be checked prior to performing a biopsy, in particular any risk of infective endocarditis (see Appendix) or prolonged bleeding. Although probably a theoretical problem rather than a major risk, a history of previous systemic steroid therapy (within the past two years) may necessitate the need for steroid cover to prevent patient collapse. In young children or the mentally handicapped, co-operation may be difficult to obtain and therefore the biopsy may have to be performed under general anaesthesia.

A decision to perform either an incisional or excisional biopsy is usually determined

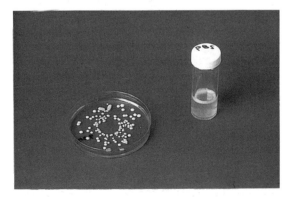

Figure 4.2 Rinse and incubated spiral plate

by the nature and size of the lesion being investigated. A small localized lesion can be simply removed (excisional biopsy), whereas with large areas of mucosal disease, it is only possible to sample a representative area (incisional biopsy).

One of the first decisions that has to be made concerns the selection of local anaesthesia. Lignocaine (2%) with adrenaline (1:80 000) is the agent of choice. The use of prilocaine (3%) with felypressin (0.03 iu/ml) has been suggested for patients with a history of hyperthyroidism, hypertension or antidepressant drug therapy but the potential problems with use of adrenaline in these patients is probably more theoretical than actual. When primary wound closure is not possible, as occurs in palatal biopsies, the use of an adhesive dressing or pack is recommended to achieve tissue coverage and haemostasis. Instruments and supplies for routine mucosal biopsy are listed in Table 4.6 and the methodology of the procedure is outlined in Table 4.7 and Plates 1 (a–f).

Medium-sized (3/0 or 4/0) black silk, on a cutting 15 mm curved needle, is the suture of choice for closure after most mucosal biopsies. A monofilament suture material (4/0–6/0) should be used to close any area of skin involved. If a general anaesthetic has been necessary to obtain a biopsy, a resorbable suture (polyglycolic acid) is recommended. Resorbable sutures are also useful

Table 4.6 Instruments and supplies for mucosal biopsy

Syringe
Needle
Local anaesthetic
Scalpel holder
Scalpel blade
Toothed tissue tweezers
Artery forceps
Dental probe
Suction tips
Sutures
Needle holder
Suture scissors

Table 4.7 Procedure for mucosal biopsy

1. Infiltration anaesthesia
2. Placement of suture (preferable to the use of tissue tweezers)
3. Lower incision
4. Upper incision
5. Separation of biopsy tissue
6. Placement of tissue on filter paper
7. Placement of biopsy in formalin (or on ice for frozen section)
8. Suture
9. Postoperative instruction
10. Arrange review

for patients who are unable to return within 1 week for review.

Biopsy tissue is routinely fixed in a formal saline. The volume of fixative into which the specimen is placed should be at least ten times the volume of the specimen. The biopsy material should be laid, connective tissue down, on a piece of filter paper and allowed to dry for 10–30 seconds prior to placement in the fixative. This will enable the laboratory to process the specimen more easily because it will minimize distortion of the specimen. The specimen jar should be labelled and the request form completed in full.

Some consideration should be given to which laboratory the specimen should be sent to. Although general pathologists have a wide range of experience they may not have a great expertise in oral disease, and it is therefore preferable to send specimens to a specialist oral pathology unit. Material of unusual cases may subsequently be submitted to specialist units or national advisory groups for interpretation.

Cytology

A cytological smear can be obtained by scraping the surface of a lesion with a wooden spatula or flat metal instrument and spreading the collected material evenly over a glass slide. Alternatively, material can be collected with a variety of brushes designed for cervical smears and transferred to a glass slide directly or following centrifugation. Although exfoliative cytology has a role in the investigation of precancer and cancer of the cervix in women at the present time it has limited use in the diagnosis of squamous cell carcinoma in the mouth. However, this method of collecting a sample of the epithelium is pain free and may have a useful role of monitoring dysplastic changes in the future if the technique can be improved.

Aspiration biopsy

Soft tissue lesions can be sampled by aspiration with a wide-bore needle (not less than 14 gauge). Such investigation is simple and extremely useful in determining whether an abnormality is solid or contains pus, cystic fluid or blood.

Frozen section

There are two main reasons for undertaking frozen-section analysis; either for rapid diagnosis of malignancy or for performance of direct immunofluorescence. A biopsy for frozen section (again placed on filter paper) should be placed on to dry ice and sent to the laboratory with an appropriate request form. The laboratory should be notified in advance that frozen material is being sent.

Table 4.8 Role of immunofluorescence studies in oral disease

Disease	Mucosal involvement	Direct immunofluorescence	Indirect immunofluorescence
Intraepithelial bullae			
Pemphigus vulgaris	Yes	Intercellular IgG and C_3	Positive
Pemphigus vegetans	Usually		Positive
Pemphigus foliaceus	No		Positive
Herpes simplex	Yes	Negative	Negative
Herpes zoster	Yes	Negative	Negative
Familial benign chronic pemphigus	Yes	Negative	Negative
Subepithelial bullae			
Epidermolysis bullosa	Yes (in dystrophic type)	Negative	Negative
Bullous pemphigoid	Yes	Linear IgG and C_3 at the basement membrane zone	Positive
Mucous membrane pemphigoid	Yes	Linear IgG and C_3 at the basement membrane zone	Variable
Dermatitis herpetiformis	Yes	Granular IgA at base of rete ridges	Negative
Lichen planus	Yes	Negative	Negative
Lichenoid eruption	Yes	Negative	May be positive giving 'string of pearls' effect
Erythema multiforme	Yes	No	Negative
Linear IgA disease	Yes	Linear IgA at the basement membrane zone	Negative

Adapted from Lamey, P-J. and Lewis, M.A.O. (1985) *Dental Update* **12**, 580

The advantage of having a frozen section result within an hour can be outweighed by the disadvantage that it is difficult, if not impossible, to assess epithelial dysplasia with confidence in tissue sections prepared from such material. Thus a frozen section may be used to exclude the presence of carcinoma at the time of surgical resection, but it does not have a role in the initial diagnosis of mucosal lesions within the mouth.

Immunofluorescence (IF) studies are indicated in patients who are suspected of having vesiculobullous disorders, such as pemphigus vulgaris, (benign) mucous membrane pemphigoid or linear IgA disease. If possible an area of mucosa including intact or recently ruptured bullae should be obtained. Many laboratories prefer that a clotted 10 ml sample of venous blood from the patient accompanies the frozen material to examine for circulating antibodies. Direct immunofluorescence investigation involves the use of an antibody to human immunoglobulin (raised in an animal) and a second antibody to the appropriate animal immunoglobulin, tagged with the fluorescent dye fluorescein. In indirect immunofluorescence the patient's serum can be applied to reference tissue such as human vagina or oesophagus to determine the presence of circulating autoantibodies to squamous cell epithelium. The value of direct and indirect immunofluorescence studies in the diagnosis of vesiculobullous disorders is outlined in Table 4.8.

4.11 Imaging techniques

Radiography

Radiographs provide useful information on orofacial conditions which have a tooth or osseous involvement. Intraoral films are used to demonstrate changes in the teeth or alveolar bone and the presence of submandibular calculi or unerupted teeth. Extraoral radiographs are used to detect abnormalities within the facial bones and skull.

An orthopantomogram is a useful and convenient radiological technique which provides a view of the entire mandible and most of the maxilla. It is not possible in this text to include details of the numerous techniques of orofacial radiography and the reader is referred to the further reading section. Radiographic examination of the salivary glands using radio-opaque contrast media (sialography) is discussed in Chapter 18.

Contrast media can also be introduced, under local anaesthesia, into the lower joint space of the temporomandibular joint; a technique known as arthrography.

Radiographs should only be taken when it is felt that the films will provide essential information, due to the potential hazard of cumulative radiation for the patient. There is no place for multiple or repeated taking of radiographs. It is good practice to make copy films when referring patients for a further opinion or treatment.

Computed tomography (CT)

Computed tomography measures variations in tissue radiodensity and allows both hard and soft structures to be examined. In addition, CT can be used to detect abnormalities at sites which would be difficult to visualize using standard radiographs.

Magnetic resonance imaging (MRI)

This method of body imaging has the major advantage over radiography and tomography in that it employs high frequency electric waves and magnetic field changes rather than ionizing radiation. Although the role of MRI in the diagnosis of orofacial disease has not been established, it has been used to detect abnormalities of the temporomandibular joints and salivary glands. It is likely to be used more extensively in the future.

Isotopic scanning

Radioactive isotopes can be used to demonstrate the presence of inflammatory and neoplastic disorders of the salivary glands and bone. The technique makes use of the preferential update of isotopes which emit gamma radiation by certain tissues. This uptake can then be detected using a gamma camera. Such investigation, using pertechnetate, is useful in determining salivary gland function (salivary scintiscanning) and this is discussed in more detail in Chapter 18.

Further reading

Goaz, P. W. and White, S. C. (1987) *Oral Radiography. Principles and Interpretation*, The CV Mosby Company, St Louis

MacFarlane, T. W. and Samaranayake, L. P. (1989) *Clinical Oral Microbiology*, Wright, London

Samaranayake, L. P., MacFarlane, T. W., Lamey, P-J. and Ferguson, M. M. (1986) A comparison of oral rinse and imprint sampling techniques for the detection of yeast, coliform and *Staphylococcus aureus* in the oral cavity. *Journal of Oral Pathology*, **15**, 386–388

Smith, N. J. D. (1988) *Dental Radiography*, 2nd ed, Blackwell Scientific Publications, Oxford

Part Three

Diseases of the Oral Mucosa

Chapter 5
Infection

The oral cavity is inhabited by a complex mixture of microorganisms that comprise the commensal oral microflora. This microflora usually contains bacteria, mycoplasma, fungi and protozoa, all of which may produce symptomatic opportunistic infection depending on local factors or reduced host defence. In addition, a number of viruses may either cause orofacial lesions or be present asymptomatically within saliva at times of acute systemic viral infection or in healthy carriers.

5.1 Bacterial infection

Endogenous bacteria are primarily involved in the two most common human diseases, namely periodontal disease and dental caries. Although rare, the infective conditions tuberculosis, gonorrhoea and syphilis can affect the oral mucosa and it is important to be able to recognize them.

Tuberculosis

At one time secondary infection of the oral mucosa by *Mycobacterium tuberculosis* within the sputum of patients with active pulmonary tuberculosis was common. Oral tuberculosis is now extremely rare in Europe and North America, although there is an increased incidence in patients with AIDS. The intraoral lesions usually form on the dorsal surface of the tongue but may affect any site.

Diagnosis

Mucosal biopsy should be undertaken and examined for tubercle follicles. Ziehl-Neelsen staining may show tubercle bacilli but this is exceptional and therefore part of any biopsy should be sent for microbiological culture. It is important to inform the laboratory that tuberculosis is suspected because specialized media (Lowenstein-Jensen's) and prolonged incubation (2–3 months) is required for isolation of the organism. A Mantoux test should be positive as a result of previous infection.

Management

Localized treatment is not required because oral lesions will resolve when systemic chemotherapy, such as rifampicin, isoniazid or ethambutol, is administered.

Gonorrhoea

This sexually transmitted disease has reached epidemic proportions in some countries and oral involvement is being diagnosed with increasing frequency in sexually active adults, especially male homosexuals. The lesions usually represent primary infection and arise as a result of orogenital contact. The patient will complain of a painful oral mucosa accompanied by altered taste, halitosis and lymphadenopathy. Clinical examination may reveal a variety of signs, including erythema, oedema, ulceration and pseudomembranes, particularly in the tonsillar region or oropharynx.

Diagnosis

Swabs of lesions should be placed in Stewart's transport medium and sent to the laboratory immediately for microscopy and culture.

Management

Treatment of gonorrhoea is based on the provision of systemic antibiotic therapy, the first choice being procaine penicillin, given either intramuscularly on its own or orally in combination with probenecid.

Syphilis

Although the primary lesion of this venereal disease usually occurs on the genital area it can present on the lips or oral mucosa, usually as a result of orogenital contact.

The primary lesion of acquired syphilis is characterized by the development of a firm nodule which breaks down after a few days to leave a painless ulcer with indurated margins. Cervical lymph nodes are usually enlarged and rubbery in consistency. The primary lesion (chancre) is highly infectious and therefore should be examined with extreme caution. Primary syphilis usually resolves within 8–9 weeks without scarring.

Secondary syphilis appears clinically approximately 6 weeks after the primary infection and is characterized by a macular or papular rash, febrile illness, malaise, headache, generalized lymphadenopathy and sore throat. The mucosa is involved in approximately one-third of patients and the lesions are described as 'snail track ulcers'. Secondary syphilis will resolve within 2–6 weeks.

Syphilis may become latent and produce tertiary lesions many years after initial infection. Fortunately, lesions of tertiary syphilis are rarely seen in the UK now, due to the successful treatment of earlier stages. Two lesions recognized as signs of tertiary syphilis are a gumma in the palate and leukoplakia affecting the dorsal surface of the tongue.

Diagnosis

Diagnosis is supported if a smear taken from either primary or secondary lesions (examined by dark-field microscopy) reveals numerous spirochaetes in size and form typical of *Treponema pallidum*. However, serological investigations (10 ml clotted sample) are the most reliable way of diagnosing syphilis from the late stage of primary infection onwards because *Treponema pallidum* cannot be routinely cultured *in vitro*. Venereal diseases reference laboratory (VDRL), *Treponema pallidum* haemagglutination (TPHA) and fluorescent treponema antibody absorbed (FTA abs) tests should be undertaken.

Treatment

The most effective treatment of any stage of syphilis is with intramuscular procaine penicillin. Patients should be followed up for at least two years and serological examination repeated over this period of time.

5.2 Fungal infection

Although a variety of fungi may cause orofacial disease, the vast majority of fungal conditions are due to *Candida* species.

Candidosis

Approximately 40% of the population harbour candidal species intraorally in small numbers as part of their normal oral microflora. Oral candidosis has been described as 'the disease of the diseased' because it often indicates underlying illness which allows proliferation of the candidal component of the oral flora. The spectrum of *Candida* species which can form in the oral cavity includes *Candida albicans*, *Candida glabrata*, *Candida tropicalis*, *Candida pseudotropicalis*, *Candida guillerimondi* and *Candida krusei*.

Table 5.1 Predisposing factors to oral candidosis

Infancy	Iron deficiency
Old age	Vitamin B_{12} deficiency
Pregnancy	Undiagnosed or poorly
Mucosal irritation	controlled diabetes
Denture wearing	mellitus
Drug therapy	Hypothyroidism
Antibiotics	Leukaemia
Corticosteroids	Agranulocytosis
Immunosuppressives	HIV infection
Cytotoxics	Xerostomia
Malnutrition	High carbohydrate diet

Although any candidal species can cause oral infection, the vast majority of cases are due to *Candida albicans*. A number of predisposing factors have been implicated in the development of oral candidosis (Table 5.1).

Oral candidosis is often categorized into five sub-groups (Table 5.2). However, concern has been expressed over the use of the term 'atrophic' to describe an area of mucosa infected with candida which may appear erythematous due to increased vascularity rather than reduced thickness of the epithelium. In addition, it is now recognized that pseudomembranous candidiosis may be a

Table 5.2 Classification of candidal infection (Group I) confined to oral and perioral tissues (primary oral candidosis)

Subgroup	Current nomenclature	Synonym	Subgroup	Revised nomenclature*
1	Acute pseudomembranous	Thrush	1	Acute pseudomembranous
2	Acute atrophic	Candidal glossitis or antibiotic sore mouth	2	Acute erythematous
3	Chronic hyperplastic	Candidal leukoplakia	3	Chronic plaque-like
			4	Chronic nodular†
4	Chronic atrophic	Denutre-induced stomatitis or denture-sore mouth	5	Chronic erythematous
		—	6	Chronic pseudomembranous†
5	Acute or chronic angular cheilitis	Perlèche	7	*Candida*-associated angular cheilitis

*Adapted from Samaranayake, L.P. and MacFarlane, T.W. (1990) *Oral Candidosis*. Wright, London
†New subdivision

Table 5.3 Classification of candidal infection (group II) when involvement of the oral and perioral tissues is accompanied by generalized or systemic candidosis

Subgroup	Condition
1	Familial chronic mucocutaneous candidosis
2	Diffuse chronic mucocutaneous candidosis
3	Candidosis-endocrinopathy syndrome
4	Familial mucocutaneous candidosis
5a	Severe combined immunodeficiency
5b	Di-George's syndrome
5c	Chronic granulomatous disease
6	Acquired immunodeficiency syndrome (AIDS)

Table 5.4 Antifungal agents used for the treatment of oral and perioral candidosis

Drug	Format
Amphotericin	Oral suspension 100 mg/ml
	Ointment 3%
	Lozenge 10 mg
	Tablet 100 mg
Nystatin	Cream 100 000 units/g
	Ointment 100 000 units/g
	Pastille 100 000 units
	Oral suspension 100 000 units/ml
Miconazole	Oral gel 25 mg/ml
	Cream 2%
	Tablets 250 mg
Fluconazole	Capsule 50 mg and 150 mg
Itraconazole	Capsule 100 mg

chronic condition, particularly in immuno-compromised patients. A new classification involving seven sub-types has recently been proposed (Table 5.2).

As well as isolated oral candidoses, candidal infection can occur in the mouth as part of a mucocutaneous candidosis (Table 5.3). In these conditions infection develops at sites such as the nails, eyes, pharynx and scalp. Mucocutaneous disorders are uncommon and therefore will not be described in detail in this text.

Management

Although management of oral candidosis will depend on the type of candidosis present, it is essential to exclude the possibility of any predisposing factors (Table 5.1). In the past, therapy has been based on the use of the polyene agents, amphotericin or nystatin, both of which are available in a variety of formulations for topical use (Table 5.4). In recent years systemic imidazole agents have been developed. One of the first of these was ketoconazole which, although safer than systemic amphotericin, is hepatotoxic. The new generation of imidazole derivatives includes fluconazole and itraconazole, both

of which appear to be extremely effective. The development of these agents is likely to represent a major advance in the management of oral candidosis.

Acute pseudomembranous candidosis (thrush)

This form of oral candidosis is characterized by soft creamy-yellow patches which may affect large areas of the oral mucosa (Plate 2). These plaques are not adherent and can usually be wiped off to reveal an underlying erythematous mucosa. Age is an important factor in the development of oral candidosis because thrush affects approximately 5% of newborn infants and 10% of elderly debilitated individuals. Thrush occurring in adulthood is usually either due to the presence of an underlying disorder, such as sideropenia, blood dyscrasias or HIV infection, or secondary to antibiotic or steroid drug therapy.

Diagnosis

A smear of thrush should be taken and stained (Gram's stain or periodic acid-Schiff reagent) to demonstrate large numbers of fungal hyphae or blastospores. A swab and oral rinse should also be taken and sent for culture.

Management

Topical polyene therapy should produce resolution within 7–10 days. Therapy should be continued for 2 weeks after clinical resolution, which in practical terms means a total of 4 weeks' application.

Acute erythematous (atrophic) candidosis

As the name implies, the oral mucosa in this form of candidosis is erythematous (Plate 3). Predisposing factors are antibiotic therapy, steroid therapy and HIV infection. Any site of the oral mucosa may be affected, but involvement of the palate and the dorsal surface of the tongue is frequently seen in patients on steroid inhaler therapy. Unlike other forms of oral candidosis, acute erythematous candidosis is often painful.

Diagnosis

A smear, swab and oral rinse should be taken and sent for culture.

Management

Topical polyene therapy should be given for 4 weeks. Antibiotic therapy should be avoided and patients on steroid inhaler therapy should be advised to rinse/gargle with water after inhaler therapy to minimize persistence of steroid in the oral cavity.

Chronic plaque-like/nodular (hyperplastic) candidosis

Chronic candidal infection can cause hyperplastic epithelial changes which present clinically as speckled white patches (Plate 4). Although this form of candidosis can occur at any intraoral site, it characteristically presents bilaterally in the commissure region of the buccal mucosa. This form of oral candidosis, particularly at the commissure site, has occasionally been associated with severe dysplasia or malignant transformation.

Diagnosis

A scraping and oral rinse should be taken and sent for culture. In addition, a mucosal biopsy of an area of affected mucosa which has not been swabbed should be performed. Histological examination should reveal the presence of candidal hyphae within a hyperplastic epithelium accompanied by a characteristic inflammatory reaction.

Management

Prolonged (up to 3 months) antifungal therapy in the form of topical polyene agents is advised. More recently, the use of systemic antifungal agents has been found to produce clinical and histological resolution in 2–3 weeks. Any iron deficiency or underlying disease should be treated.

Chronic erythematous (atrophic) candidosis

This is the form of oral candidosis most frequently seen and it affects between a quarter and two-thirds of patients who wear dentures (Plate 5). Continuous coverage of the palatal mucosa is a recognized predisposing factor to chronic erythematous candidosis, and clearly the habit of wearing dentures both day and night should be discouraged. In addition, the disease is not infrequent beneath the mucosal coverage area of upper orthodontic appliances.

Diagnosis

Separate smears and swabs should be taken from areas of affected mucosa and the fitting surface of dentures. The smears will reveal numerous fungal forms along with occasional leukocytes. In addition to swabs an oral rinse should be sent for culture.

Management

Management is with topical polyene anti-fungal agents, given 6-hourly for 4 weeks. In this group of patients adequate denture hygiene is also important. Patients should therefore be advised to soak acrylic prostheses in a dilute solution of hypochlorite overnight to eliminate any candidal infestation of dentures. Patients who have upper dentures made of cobalt chromium should soak their dentures overnight in chlorhexidine (0.2%).

Candida-associated angular cheilitis

Angular cheilitis is a common condition which presents as inflammation at either one or both corners of the mouth (Plate 6). It may be associated with any form of intraoral candidosis. *Candida* species can be isolated from approximately two-thirds of patients with angular cheilitis, either alone or in combination with staphylococci or streptococci. Colonization of the angles of the mouth with candida is probably a result of direct spread of the organisms from the oral flora, whilst colonization with staphylococcal species is known by phage typing to be due to spread from the anterior nares.

Diagnosis

Separate smears and swabs should be taken from each angle of the mouth, each anterior nares, the palate and (if worn) fitting-surface of upper denture. An oral rinse should also be sent for culture.

Management

Management is by eradication of the chronic reservoir of candidal infection. Patients should therefore be provided with topical polyene antifungal agents (6-hourly for 4 weeks) and advised on denture hygiene. If staphylococci alone are isolated from both the angles and anterior nares then fucidic acid or mupirocin cream should be prescribed for use 6-hourly for a 4-week period. Two tubes of either agent should be issued to the patient, who is instructed to use one tube exclusively for the angles and the other for the anterior nares.

Other mycoses

A number of rare forms of systemic mycosis can produce orofacial lesions. Such conditions include paracoccidiodomycosis, histoplasmosis, and mucormycosis. However, it is not possible to cover these conditions in a text of this size.

5.3 Viral infection

Many viruses can produce oral and perioral disease. Several viruses, such as the herpes group, cause erosion or ulceration, but others, such as human papilloma virus, may cause mucosal overgrowths. Current research is aimed at elucidating the role of viruses in a variety of oral diseases, including lichen planus and squamous cell carcinoma. In addition, paramyxovirus and Epstein-Barr virus have been implicated in disorders of the salivary glands.

The Herpes group of viruses

This group of viruses, which comprises *Herpes simplex* type I, *Herpes simplex* type II, *Varicella zoster*, Epstein-Barr virus and cytomegalovirus, account for the majority of virally-induced oral mucosal lesions.

Primary herpetic gingivostomatitis

Primary herpetic gingivostomatitis is one of the most common viral infections that affects the oral cavity. Approximately 60% of adults have evidence of previous infection in the form of antibody by the age of 16 years. This condition has traditionally been attributed to infection with *Herpes simplex* virus type I, but it is now recognized that *Herpes simplex* virus type II, which was previously associated only with genital herpetic lesions, may also be involved. The severity of clinical symptoms is variable and it is likely that the vast majority of primary infections go unnoticed or are dismissed as teething during childhood. However, it has been estimated that approximately 5% of individuals who encounter the virus develop significant symptoms which include oral ulceration, coated tongue, pyrexia and cervical lymphadenopathy (Plate 7).

Diagnosis

Clinical presentation is usually diagnostic, however, confirmation can be made by demonstration of a four-fold rise in serological antibody titre or isolation of virus in tissue culture. Clinical kits, based on the use of immunofluorescence, have recently become available and these can rapidly detect the presence of *Herpes simplex* virus.

Treatment

Patients and/or their parents should be reassured about the basis of the condition and advised of the infectious nature of the lesions. Instructions should be given to limit touching affected areas of the lips and mouth to reduce the risk of the spread of infection to other sites. Acyclovir, an antiviral agent effective against *Herpes simplex*, should be instituted in severe cases. The standard regime is a 200 mg tablet or 5 ml suspension 5-times daily for 5 days. This dosage should be halved in children under the age of 2 years. Supportive symptomatic therapy, such as chlorhexidine mouthwashes, analgesic therapy, soft diet and encouraging fluid intake, are also important factors in management.

Recurrent Herpes simplex infection

Recurrent *Herpes simplex* infection typically causes herpes labialis (Plate 8). The symptoms of herpes labialis (prodromal stage) begin as a pricking or burning sensation on one area of the lips. Within 24 hours a vesicle develops which ruptures within a further 48 hours to leave an erosive area of epithelium which subsequently crusts over and heals. Factors which may predispose to the development of herpes labialis in susceptible individuals include sunlight, trauma, stress, fever, menstruation and immunosuppression.

Although herpes labialis is a well-recognized entity indicative of *Herpes simplex* reactivation, there is evidence that the virus can also produce recurrent intraoral ulceration. As with herpes labialis, the patient with intraoral herpes is usually aware of prodromal tingling. The mucosa of the hard palate is the site most commonly involved, but other areas, such as the lower buccal sulcus, can also be affected. It can be difficult to deduce whether the lesion(s) were precipitated by trauma in these patients or whether they chronically shed *Herpes simplex* virus in their saliva which subsequently colonizes traumatized mucosa.

Diagnosis

The clinical appearance is usually diagnostic. Confirmation can be made by isolation of the virus in tissue culture or the use of immunofluorescence on a smear of a recent lesion.

Treatment

In many cases no active treatment is indicated, but the patient should be warned about the infectivity of the lesion. The use of acyclovir in the prodromal phase may be effective in aborting herpes labialis.

Varicella zoster

Primary infection with *Varicella zoster* virus causes chickenpox, whereas subsequent reactivation of the virus produces shingles (herpes zoster).

Chickenpox, a common infectious disease of childhood, is characterized by the appearance of a maculopapular skin rash. Typically, lesions arise on the trunk and spread to the face and limbs. This is opposite to the spread of infection found in measles. In many patients with chickenpox the cutaneous lesions may be preceded or accompanied by small (2–4 mm diameter) oral ulcers in the palate and faucial region.

Reactivation of latent *Varicella zoster* virus in sensory nerve ganglia produces severe pain which is followed by vesiculobullous cutaneous or mucosal lesions similar to those due to *Herpes simplex* (Plate 9). The trigeminal nerve is affected in about 15% of cases of shingles, usually with one division (ophthalmic, maxillary or mandibular) being involved. Lesions are characteristically unilateral and limited to the sensory innervation of one division of the nerve. The lesions of shingles may heal with scarring and show a degree of post-inflammatory pigmentation as well as residual sensory dysfunction.

Diagnosis

Clinical presentation is often so characteristic that diagnosis is made easily. Confirmation of the disease can be made by virus isolation in cell culture or immunofluorescence on a smear from a recent lesion.

Treatment

Chickenpox does not usually require any treatment, although bed rest and patient isolation are advised during the active phase of the disease. Before the development of acyclovir, the treatment of shingles was limited to either topical antiviral therapy or analgesics for relief of pain. Ideally, treatment (800 mg tablet of acyclovir, 5 times daily for 7–10 days) should be instituted as early as possible, preferably before the development of vesicles. Post-herpetic neuralgia may be a problem in these patients, and it is thought that a 10-day course of acyclovir therapy may limit this complication.

Ramsay-Hunt syndrome

This condition is generally accepted to be infection of the geniculate ganglion involving *Varicella zoster* virus. The syndrome consists of facial nerve palsy, vesicular eruptions on the external auditory meatus and ulceration of the mucosa in the oropharynx. Auditory dysfunction in the form of hyperacusis results from involvement of the stapedius muscle.

Diagnosis

Clinical presentation is usually diagnostic.

Treatment

It is treated with acyclovir in a full 10-day herpes zoster regime and systemic steroids. The normal precautions when prescribing systemic steroids apply. In practice reasonably high doses of prednisolone (up to 40 mg daily in a decreasing dose over 3 weeks) are employed to encourage resolution of the facial nerve palsy.

Coxsackie virus infections

The Coxsackie viruses are subdivided into group A and group B. Several viruses can produce painful orofacial conditions, including hand, foot and mouth disease and herpangina. Hand, foot and mouth disease is usually caused by Coxsackie virus A16 but may also be due to infection with types A4, A5, A9 and A10. As the name of the condition implies, the distribution of lesions is characteristic, involving macular and vesicular eruptions on the hands, feet and mucosa of the pharynx, soft palate, buccal sulcus or tongue. Symptoms usually resolve within 7–10 days. The cutaneous lesions of hand, foot and mouth disease are transient, lasting only 1–3 days, and may be asymptomatic. There is little or no systemic upset in the disease.

Herpangina is due to infection by Coxsackie virus A2, A4, A5, A6 or A8. This condition occurs predominantly in children and presents as sudden onset of fever and sore throat with subsequent development of papular, vesicular lesions on the oral mucosa and pharyngeal mucosa. The severity of symptoms is variable, but clinical resolution usually occurs within 7–10 days even in the absence of treatment.

Diagnosis

Clinical appearance is usually diagnostic. Viral culture for Coxsackie infections is not widely available, and therefore diagnosis is based on demonstration of increased convalescent antibody levels.

Treatment

Bed rest and the use of antiseptic mouthwash are advised. Patients should be encouraged to maintain adequate fluid intake.

Epstein-Barr virus

Epstein-Barr virus is the usual cause of infectious mononucleosis, which is characterized by lymph node enlargement, fever and pharyngeal inflammation. Approximately 30% of patients will also suffer from purpura or petechiae in the palate and oral ulceration. Occasionally gingival bleeding and ulceration resembling acute necrotizing ulcerative gingivitis may develop. The condition occurs mainly in childhood or early adolescence and is believed to be transmitted via saliva.

Diagnosis

Serological demonstration of IgM antibody to Epstein-Barr virus capsid antigen and a positive Monospot slide test or Paul-Bunnell (Davidson) test will confirm a diagnosis of infectious mononucleosis.

Treatment

No specific treatment is required, although hospitalization may be necessary in severe cases of infectious mononucleosis with hepatic or splenic involvement. Penicillin therapy should be avoided since it is likely to produce an erythematous skin rash.

Human papillomavirus

To date, more than 65 distinct types of human papillomavirus (HPV) have been identified. This group of DNA viruses has been implicated in the development of hyperplastic papillomatous and verrucous squamous cell lesions in the skin and various mucosal sites. Conditions occurring within the mouth that have been suggested to be related to HPV infection include focal epithelial hyperplasia (Heck's disease), squamous papilloma, condyloma accuminatum, verruca vulgaris, leukoplakia and squamous cell carcinoma. It must be emphasized, however, that involvment of HPV in these lesions is not yet proved and further research work is presently being undertaken to establish the role of this virus in oral disease.

Further reading

Cawson, R. A. (1986) An update on antiviral therapy: the advent of acyclovir. *British Dental Journal*, **161**, 245–252

Lamey, P-J., Lewis, M. A. O. (1989) Oral medicine in practice: viral infection. *British Dental Journal*, **167**, 269–274

Lamey, P-J., Lewis, M. A. O. and MacDonald, D. G. (1989) Treatment of candidal leukoplakia with fluconazole. *British Dental Journal* **166**, 296–298

Lamey, P-J., Lewis, M. A. O., Rennie, J. S. and Beattie, A. D. (1990) Heck's disease. *British Dental Journal*, **168**, 251–252

Lewis, M. A. O., Meechan, C. MacFarlane, T. W., Lamey, P-J. and Kay, E. J. (1989) Presentation and antimicrobial treatment of orofacial infections in general dental practice. *British Dental Journal*, **161**, 41–45

Lewis, M. A. O., Samaranayake, L. P. and Lamey, P-J. (1991) Diagnosis and treatment of oral candidosis. *Journal of Oral Maxillofacial Surgery* **49**, 996–1002

MacFarlane, T. W. and Samaranayake, L. P. (1989) *Clinical Oral Microbiology*, Wright, London.

MacFarlane, T. W. and Helnarska, S. J. (1968) The microbiology of angular cheilitis. *British Dental Journal* **140**, 403–406

MacFarlane, T. W. and Samaranayake, L. P. (1990) Systemic infections. In *Oral manifestations of Systemic Disease* (eds J. H. Jones and D. K. Mason), Baillière Tindall, London, pp. 339–386

McCracken, A. W. and Cawson, R. A. (1983) *Clinical and Oral Microbiology*, Hemisphere Publishing Corporation, London

Samaranayake, L. P. (1991) Superficial oral fungal infections. *Current Opinion in Dentistry*, **1**, 415–422

Samaranayake, L. P. and MacFarlane, T. W. (1990) *Oral Candidosis*, Wright, Bristol

Scully, C., Epstein, J., Porter, S. and Cox, M. (1991) Viruses and chronic disorders involving the human oral mucosa. *Oral Surgery, Oral Medicine, Oral Pathology*, **72**, 537–544

Chapter 6
Ulceration

6.1 Trauma	6.3 Behçet's disease
6.2 Recurrent aphthous stomatitis	6.4 Acute necrotizing ulcerative gingivitis

Many patients suffer from oral ulceration and they frequently seek help due to the pain. Common causes of oral ulceration include trauma, recurrent aphthous stomatitis, mucocutaneous diseases (Chapter 9), bacterial infections (Chapter 5), viral infections (Chapter 5), haemapoetic disease and deficiency states (Chapter 11) and squamous cell carcinoma (Chapter 8).

6.1 Trauma

Traumatic causes of oral ulceration may be physical or chemical. Physical damage to the oral mucosa may be caused by sharp surfaces, such as clasps or peripheral borders of dentures, orthodontic appliances, cheek biting habits or fractured teeth. Oral ulceration caused during seizures is well-recognized in poorly controlled epileptics. Rarely, oral ulceration may be self-induced (stomatitis artefacta) in the same way that some patients deliberately cause skin lesions in dermatitis artefacta.

Chemical irritation of the oral mucosa may produce ulceration. A common cause of this type of injury is placement of aspirin tablets or toothache creams adjacent to painful teeth or under uncomfortable dentures.

Diagnosis

Traumatic ulceration characteristically presents as a single irregular ulcer. Often the cause of trauma becomes obvious from the history or clinical examination.

Management

Whenever trauma is suspected as the likely aetiological factor, the cause should be eliminated and the patient provided with an antiseptic mouthwash such as chlorhexidine. If the lesion is truly traumatic in origin it should heal within 7–10 days. Any ulcer persisting beyond this time should be biopsied to exclude carcinoma. Any patient suspected of deliberately self-inducing injury (artefacting) should be challenged with this and the general medical practitioner informed.

6.2 Recurrent aphthous stomatitis

Recurrent aphthous stomatitis (RAS) is one of the most common mucosal disorders and affects approximately 15–20% of the population in the UK at some time. Higher prevalences have been found in upper socio-economic groups and among students at the times of examinations.

Several classifications of RAS have been proposed, but on clinical grounds the condition may be divided into three sub-types; minor, major and herpetiform. All types of ulceration are associated with pain.

Most (80%) patients with RAS suffer from the minor form (MiRAS), which is characterized by round or oval shallow ulcers less than 5 mm in diameter surrounded by an erythematous border (Plate 10). Ulceration in MiRAS tends to affect the non-keratinized sites, such as labial mucosa, buccal mucosa and floor of mouth. Ulcers are either single or in crops of four or five and heal within 10–14 days without scarring.

Major recurrent aphthous stomatitis (MaRAS), which accounts for approximately 10% of patients with RAS, is more severe than that seen in MiRAS. Classically, the ulcers are approximately 1–3 cm in diameter, last for 4 weeks or more and can affect any site of the oral mucosa including keratinized sites (Plate 11). Evidence of previous ulcers can often be seen in patients with MaRAS; scarring is due to the severity and prolonged nature of the lesions.

The third and least common type of RAS is herpetiform ulceration (HU). The term 'herpetiform' has been suggested because the clinical appearance of HU (which may involve as many as 100 small ulcers at any time) is similar to that of primary herpetic gingivostomatitis (Plate 12), but herpes viruses have no aetiological role in HU or indeed in any form of aphthous ulceration.

Although three clinical variants of RAS are now recognized it is still unclear if they are variants of one disease or represent different disorders which manifest as recurrent oral

Table 6.1 Proposed aetiological factors for recurrent aphthous stomatitis (RAS)

Factor	Evidence
Deficiency	Occurrence of iron, folic acid, vitamins B_{12} or B-complex deficiency
Psychology	Increased incidence of RAS in student populations prior to examinations
Trauma	Development of ulcers at sites following penetration injuries
Endocrine	Development of RAS in luteal phase of menstrual cycle in some female patients
Allergy	Raised IgE levels and association between certain foodstuffs and development of ulcers
Smoking	Development of RAS in previously asymptomatic smokers when smoking habit stopped
Hereditary	Increased incidence in children when both parents suffer RAS; high concordance between twins
Immunological	Conflicting evidence, but some information on abnormal levels of immunoglobulins

ulceration. Although many theories on the cause of RAS have been proposed (Table 6.1) no single causative factor has been identified.

Diagnosis

The diagnosis of RAS is based on clinical appearance of the ulcers and the history. Particular attention should be given to the age of onset, site, duration and frequency of ulceration. Any relationship to gastrointestinal disease, menstruation, stress and ingestion of foodstuffs should be recorded. It is important that haematological deficiency is excluded, and therefore patients should undergo a full blood count and estimations of levels of vitamin B_{12}, corrected whole blood folate and ferritin (or total iron binding capacity (TIBC) serum iron). Deficiencies of vitamins B_1, B_2 and B_6 have been reported in patients with RAS, but screening for levels of these vitamins is not undertaken routinely due to the laboratory time and cost involved in the assay.

Treatment

Many agents, including vitamins, antiseptic mouthwashes, topical steroids and systemic immunomodulators, have been suggested for the treatment of RAS (Table 6.2), but few of these have any scientifically proved efficacy. A combination of vitamin B_1 (thiamine, 300 mg daily) and vitamin B_6 (pyridoxine, 50 mg 8-hourly), given for 1 month has been suggested as initial empirical management.

Table 6.2 Suggested therapies for recurrent aphthous stomatitis (RAS)

Vitamins
   Thiamine (B_1)
   Pyridoxine (B_6)
Mouthrinses
   Chlorhexidine gluconate
   Benzydamine hydrochloride
   Carbenoxolone disodium
Topical corticosteroids
   Hydrocortisone hemisuccinate
   Triamcinolone acetonide
   Fluocinonide
   Betamethasone sodium phosphate
   Betamethasone valerate
   Beclomethasone dipropionate
   Flumethasone pivalate
Antimicrobials
   Topical tetracyclines
Immunomodulators
   Levamisole
   Transfer factor
   Colchicine
   Gammaglobulins
   Dapsone
   Thalidomide
Others
   Monoamine oxidase inhibitors
   Cromoglycate

Alternatively, some patients respond well to chlorhexidine mouthwash and topical corticosteroids, such as hydrocortisone hemisuccinate (2.5 mg pellet placed adjacent to the ulcer 3 times daily) or betamethasone sodium phosphate (0.5 mg tablet dissolved in water and used as a mouthwash held over the ulcer 3 times daily). The use of anxiolytic therapy or referral for hypnotherapy may be helpful in individuals where stress is thought to be a precipitating factor. A minority of patients with RAS associate the onset of ulceration with certain foodstuffs, thus investigations of food sensitivity is indicated in these individuals.

The use of systemic agents, such as levamisole, monoamine oxidase inhibitors, thalidomide or dapsone, has been described for patients with frequent or severe oral ulceration. However, the use of these agents should be considered carefully due to doubt about their effectiveness and their known side-effects.

6.3 Behçet's disease

The clinical triad of oral ulceration, genital ulceration and uveitis was first recognized by Hippocrates but now bears the name Behçet's disease after the Turkish dermatologist's description of the disease some 50 years ago. Behçet's disease, referred to previously as Behçet's syndrome, is a multisystem condition with a range of manifestations including oral ulceration, arthritis, cardiovascular disease, thrombophlebitis, cutaneous rashes and neurological disease.

Diagnosis

Recurrent oral ulceration is an essential feature of Behçet's disease, but confusion has arisen concerning the other criteria required to fulfil a diagnosis. An international study group has recently presented a set of criteria which have been agreed for use in the future (Table 6.3). HLA typing may be of value because there is a strong association with HLA-B5.

Table 6.3 Criteria for diagnosis of Behçet's disease

Recurrent oral ulceration	Minor aphthous, major aphthous, or herpetiform ulceration which recurred at least 3 times in one 12-month period
Plus two of:	
Recurrent genital ulceration	Aphthous ulceration or scarring
Eye lesions	Anterior uveitis, posterior uveitis, or cells in vitreous on slit examination; or retinal vasculitis observed by ophthalmologist
Skin lesions	Erythema nodosum observed by physician or patient, pseudo-folliculitis, or papulopustular lesions; or acneiform nodules observed by physician in postadolescent patients not on corticosteroid treatment
Positive pathergy test	Read by physician at 24–48 h

(Findings applicable only in absence of other clinical explanations)
International Study Group for Behçet's disease. (1990) *Lancet*, **335**, 1078–1080

Treatment

Oral lesions should be managed symptomatically as for RAS. Patients with Behçet's disease may have systemic immunosuppressive therapy and this may reduce oral symptoms. Ocular involvement must be monitored carefully because progressive uveitis can lead to scarring and possible blindness.

6.4 Acute necrotizing ulcerative gingivitis

This condition is characterized by the rapid onset of painful ulceration affecting the gingival margin and interdental papillae. The patient usually has unpleasant halitosis. The exact cause of acute necrotizing ulcer-

ative gingivitis is not fully understood, but strictly anaerobic organisms, in particular spirochaetes and *Fusobacterium* species, are likely to be involved. Smoking and stress have been implicated as predisposing factors.

Diagnosis

Although the clinical appearance is characteristic, diagnosis can be confirmed rapidly by examining a Gram-stained smear of an area of ulceration. Essential microscopic features include numerous fusobacteria, medium-sized spirochaetes and acute inflammatory cells.

Treatment

In the short-term, initial management consists of oral hygiene therapy involving thorough mechanical cleaning and debridement of the affected area. The importance of local measures cannot be overemphasized, but treatment of most cases should also involve the use of a systemic antimicrobial agent. In the past, the use of hydrogen peroxide mouthwashes, both as a mechanical cleansing agent and as an oxidizing agent, has been recommended, but the benefit of such treatment is not universally accepted. At the present time, systemic metronidazole (200 mg tablet, 8-hourly) should be prescribed for 3–5 days. This approach will usually produce a dramatic improvement within 24–48 hours. However, in the long-term, hygiene therapy to prevent further gingival damage should be arranged.

Further reading

Eversole, L. R. (1988) Diseases of the oral mucous membranes. In *Perspectives on 1988 World Workshop on Oral Medicine* (eds H. D. Millard and D.K. Mason), Year Book Medical Publishers, London, pp. 79–85
Field, A. E., Rotter, E., Speechley, J. A. and Tyldesley, W. R. (1987) Clinical and haematological assessment of children with recurrent aphthous ulceration. *British Dental Journal*, **163**, 19–22

Pedersen, A. (1989) Psychologic stress and recurrent aphthous ulceration. *Journal of Oral Pathology and Medicine*, **18** 119–122

Rennie, J. S., Reade, P. C., Hay , K. D. and Scully, C. (1985) Recurrent aphthous stomatitis. *British Dental Journal*, **159**, 361–367

Santis, H. R. (1991) Aphthous stomatitis and its management. *Current Opinion in Dentistry*, **1**, 763–768

Scully, C. and Porter, S. R. (1989) Recurrent aphthous stomatitis: current concepts of aetiology , pathogenesis and management. *Journal of Oral Pathology and Medicine*, **18**, 21–27

Tyldesley, W. R. (1983) Stomatitis and recurrent oral ulceration: Is a full blood screen necessary? *British Journal of Oral Surgery*, **21**, 27–30

Wray, D. (1984) Recurrent aphthous stomatitis. *Journal of the Royal Society of Medicine*, **77**, 1–3

Chapter 7
Developmental and miscellaneous lesions

A number of developmental conditions may affect the orofacial tissues, although most are rare. Those that do occur are usually of little significance and do not require treatment other than giving reassurance about the nature of the condition. The presence of ectopic sebaceous glands, haemangiomata or prominent lingual papillae can cause cancerphobia in some patients.

7.1 Sebaceous glands (Fordyce's spots)

Sebaceous glands may occur in the oral mucous membrane and present clinically as creamy spots below the epithelium. It has been suggested that these structures arise at this site due to the inclusion of ectoderm processes during embryonic life. Although Fordyce's spots are probably present to some degree in all patients, some individuals may have numerous glands, particularly in the retromolar region and buccal mucosa. These glands also tend to become more prominent with age.

Diagnosis

Prominent sebaceous glands have a characteristic clinical appearance and diagnosis can be made easily.

Treatment

Once recognized, no active treatment is required, although it is not uncommon for elderly patients to become concerned that these structures represent oral cancer. Obviously, strong reassurance should be given to such cancerphobic patients.

7.2 Haemangioma (vascular naevus)

Neoplasia of the blood vessels is extremely uncommon, although there has been an increased incidence in recent years due to the development of Kaposi's sarcoma in HIV-positive individuals. The vast majority of malformations of blood vessels are congenital conditions referred to as haemangiomas or vascular naevi. Haemangiomata may be divided into two forms depending on the type and size of the blood vessels involved. A capillary haemangioma consists of a mass of small fine capillary vessels, whereas a cavernous angioma contains a large, thin-walled sinus. Haemangioma may occur at any intraoral site, although the tongue, lips and buccal mucosa are most frequently affected.

Diagnosis

Haemangiomata occurring in the oral soft tissues are similar to those occurring in the skin and appear as well-circumscribed, flat or raised lesions with a blue/red discoloration. Blanching of the lesion when pressure is applied to it using a glass slide can help confirm the diagnosis of the presence of a cavernous haemangioma.

Treatment

The majority of haemangiomata require no active treatment. However, prominent or nodular regions can become progressively traumatized and give rise to problems of haemorrhaging. If symptoms persist, small localized lesions can be surgically excised or treated with cryosurgery. More extensive or deep lesions require specialist management, including surgery and the possible use of sclerosing agents.

7.3 Hereditary haemorrhagic telangiectasia (Rendu-Osler-Weber disease)

This condition is an autosomal hereditary disease which is characterized by the appearance of numerous telangiectetic or angiomatous areas of skin and oral mucosa.

Diagnosis

Diagnosis is made from the family history and clinical examination.

Treatment

Treatment will depend on the extent of symptoms, but may involve the use of surgery if repeated bleeding occurs.

7.4 Fissured tongue

The fissures on the dorsal surface of the tongue may vary considerably among individuals. The term 'fissured tongue' has been used to describe the occurrence of marked fissuring. The incidence of this condition is uncertain due to differing clinical opinions on what constitutes a fissured tongue. However, it is likely that many patients have fissured tongue without symptoms. Occasionally patients may complain of discomfort on the tongue as a result of localized inflammation within the fissures.

Diagnosis

Clinical appearance is diagnostic.

Treatment

Tongue hygiene involving the use of a topical antiseptic such as chlorhexidine usually leads to resolution of any erythema or discomfort.

7.5 Geographic tongue (benign migratory glossitis, erythema migrans)

This common condition is characterized by irregular depapillated areas surrounded by pale well-demarcated margins on the dorsal surface and lateral margins of tongue (Plate 13). Such areas appear and regress over a period of a few days. The condition is relatively common and can affect any age including young children. Patients are often unaware of the presence of geographic tongue, although some individuals complain of discomfort on eating, especially hot or spicy foods.

Diagnosis

Geographic tongue can be diagnosed from clinical appearance and history. Biopsy is rarely indicated, but should be undertaken whenever a more sinister lesion is suspected.

Treatment

The patient should be reassured about the benign nature of the condition. Nutritional

deficiency should be excluded in all patients with symptomatic geographic tongue. Therefore, a full blood count and an evaluation of levels of vitamin B_{12}, corrected whole blood folate and ferritin should be undertaken. In addition, a zinc assay may be helpful because symptomatic geographic tongue has been found to respond to zinc therapy. Zinc should be given as zinc sulphate, 200 mg 8-hourly, dissolved in water and held in the mouth for approximately 3 minutes before swallowing. In some patients symptoms of geographic tongue may be psychogenic.

7.6 Median rhomboid glossitis (superficial midline glossitis)

Median rhomboid glossitis has long been considered to be a developmental abnormality associated with the tuberculum impar. This belief probably arose due to the fact that median rhomboid glossitis characteristically presents at the junction of the anterior two-thirds and posterior one-third of the tongue. However, it has been shown recently that many of these lesions contain candida.

Diagnosis

Diagnosis can be made relatively easily from the clinical appearance. Microbiological investigations should include oral rinse and swab of the tongue. Biopsy is not indicated unless there is any doubt about the initial diagnosis.

Treatment

Treatment in the past has consisted of topical antifungal therapy in the form of lozenges or pastilles, dissolved on the midline of the tongue 8-hourly for up to 3 months. Lack of patient compliance with this treatment may in part explain the poor therapeutic results. More recently, the use of systemic antifungal agents has produced encouraging results.

7.7 Coated tongue

The tongue of healthy individuals has a coating of desquamated epithelial cells, mucus, microorganisms and debris. A variety of factors, such as decreased tongue mobility, reduced salivary production, smoking or respiratory upset can lead to an increased thickness of this coating. The coating may be discoloured, especially in patients who smoke heavily.

Diagnosis

Coated tongue is diagnosed by clinical examination.

Treatment

The awareness of a coated tongue is a common cause of anxiety, and therefore reassurance is required. Effervescent mouthwashes have been found to be helpful, although best results occur following the mechanical cleaning of the tongue with a toothbrush. In extreme cases a scalpel may be used to scrape off the hyperplastic papillae. Chemical cauterization and cryotherapy have also been suggested for possible treatment, but their success has been limited.

7.8 Polyps and granulomata

A variety of lesions can be classified under a heading 'polyps' and 'granulomata' (Table 7.1) and this group forms the most common cause of localized swellings occurring on the oral mucosa. Characteristically, these lesions present as painless sessile or pedunculated

Table 7.1 Polyps and granulomata

Fibrous epulis
Fibroepithelial polyp
Pyogenic granuloma
(Pregnancy epulis)
Denture granuloma
(Denture-induced hyperplasia)
Giant cell epulis
Giant cell granuloma

swellings which can affect any intraoral site (Plate 14). The aetiology of these lesions is unknown, but it is likely that chronic minor irritation plays an important role.

Diagnosis

Although the diagnosis of types of polyp or granulomata can frequently be made on clinical examination alone, surgical removal is the treatment of choice, and therefore clinical diagnosis can be confirmed histopathologically.

The terms fibrous epulis, fibro-epithelial polyp, denture-induced hyperplasia and pyogenic granuloma are all used to describe a similar reactive condition, depending on its site, microscopic appearance and the underlying predisposing factor.

A fibrous epulis refers to a polyp occurring on the gingival margin, whereas the term fibro-epithelial polyp is usually used when other sites are affected, such as the buccal mucosa, inner aspect of the lips or lateral margins of the tongue. When involvement coincides with the periphery of a denture, the term denture-induced hyperplasia has been used. More florid inflammatory changes are sometimes present and under these circumstances the term pyogenic granuloma is used. A particular example of this condition can be seen on the gingival margin of pregnant women, when the lesion has been referred to as pregnancy epulis.

Giant cell epulis is less common than the other irritational lesions. It only occurs on the alveolar process, usually anterior to the first molars. Diagnosis is made on histopathological examination and is characterized by the presence of multinucleated giant cells in proliferating granulation tissue.

Giant cell granuloma arises within bone, but the intraoral presentation is sometimes similar to that of giant cell epulis. Differentiation between the two is important because giant cell granuloma can rapidly cause widespread bone destruction. In addition, these lesions may arise due to underlying hyperparathyroidism.

Treatment

Treatment of all types of polyp and granulomata is based on adequate surgical removal. Lesions of denture-induced granuloma will reduce quite considerably if the associated denture periphery is relieved. Following relief of the denture, any remaining tissue can be surgically removed after approximately 3–4 weeks. If giant cell epulis or giant cell granuloma is suspected then radiographs should be undertaken to determine the extent of any bone involvement. In addition, haematological investigations of serum calcium, phosphate and alkaline phosphatase should be performed.

7.9 Squamous cell papilloma

The squamous cell papilloma is a common benign epithelial neoplasm which can arise at any age and often develops on the soft palate, lateral margins of the tongue or lips (Plate 15). The clinical appearance is classically described as 'cauliflower-like' because it consists of a discrete swelling with numerous epithelial projections which are sometimes keratinized. The cause is uncertain, but involvement of papillomavirus has been suggested. Support for a viral cause is provided by the similarity in clinical appearance to the common wart (verruca vulgaris) occurring on the skin.

Diagnosis

Clinical appearance is usually sufficiently characteristic for diagnosis, but excision biopsy should be carried out.

Treatment

Histopathological examination will confirm the clinical diagnosis and exclude condyloma accuminatum, verruca vulgaris or focal epithelial hyperplasia (Heck's disease).

7.10 Exostoses

Bony exostoses may occur intraorally and present as firm swellings. The terms torus palatinus or torus mandibularis are used respectively whenever these exostoses occur either in the midline of the hard palate or on the lingual aspect of the mandible in the premolar region. These osteomata which consist of lamellae of compact bone usually occur in adult life.

Diagnosis

Diagnosis is on clinical appearance. Blood biochemistry should be undertaken to confirm normal levels of alkaline phosphatase, calcium and phosphate.

Treatment

No treatment other than reassurance is required. However, surgical reduction of large tori may be necessary if the patient has to be provided with dentures.

Further reading

MacLeod, R. I. and Soames, J. V. (1987) Epulides: a clinicopathological study of a series of 200 consecutive lesions. *British Dental Journal*, **163**, 51–53

Soames, J. V. and Southam, J. C. (1985) *Oral Pathology*, Oxford University Press, Oxford

Scully, C., Epstein, J., Porter, S. and Cox, M. (1991) Viruses and chronic disorders involving the oral mucosa. *Oral Surgery, Oral Medicine, Oral Pathology*, **72**, 537–544

Chapter 8
Premalignant conditions and tumours

8.1 Precancer	8.3 Pigmented naevus and melanotic macule
8.2 Squamous cell carcinoma	8.4 Malignant melanoma

Oral malignancy represents a great clinical challenge because the 5-year survival rate for patients with oral cancer is approximately 50% in the UK. This figure has not changed within the past century despite efforts to diagnose oral cancer at an early stage and the use of more aggressive treatment regimes. The development of oral cancer has been associated with other mucosal lesions, particularly white or red patches and, in view of this, such lesions have been regarded as precancerous conditions. A number of terms have been proposed for use in epidemiological surveys on oral premalignancy and malignancy (Table 8.1).

8.1 Precancer

Leukoplakia (white patch) and erythroplakia (red patch) are terms used to describe mucosal abnormalities of the oral mucosa that cannot be characterized as any other disease. Patients with these conditions have a greater risk of developing oral cancer than individuals with apparently normal mucosa. However, the rate of malignant change in these lesions is variable being between 2 and 50%, with erythroplakia having a worse prognosis. The clinical presentation of these conditions can vary from a minimal localized lesion to involvement of extensive areas of the oral mucosa (Plates 16 and 17).

The clinical appearance has no relationship to the presence and degree of any dysplasia. Therefore, regardless of clinical appearance, biopsy is mandatory for all patients presenting with leukoplakia or erythroplakia. Selecting a biopsy site can be a problem when extensive areas of the oral mucosa are involved. A leukoplakic patch associated with an area of erythema is a good choice. White lesions appearing in oral sites not normally subjected to irritation,

Table 8.1 Terminology applied to oral cancer and precancer

Morbidity	
Incidence	The number of new cases of oral cancer in a defined population (usually 100 000) in a given period of time (usually one year)
Prevalence	The number of cases of oral cancer in a defined population at a specified time
Frequency	Oral cancer occurring at a given site expressed as a percentage of oral cancer in all sites
Precancerous lesion	A morphologically altered tissue in which oral cancer is more likely to occur than in its apparent normal counterpart
Leukoplakia*	A white patch or plaque which cannot be characterized clinically or pathologically as any other disease
Erythroplakia*	A bright red velvet patch that cannot be characterized clinically or pathologically as being due to any other condition
Mortality	
Mortality rate	The number of deaths resulting from oral cancer in a defined population in a specified period of time

* These terms are unrelated to the absence or presence of dysplasia

Table 8.2 Initial assessment of leukoplakia or erythroplakia

History
Site
Tobacco habit
Alcohol intake
Haematological
    Full blood count
    Vitamin B_{12}
    Ferritin
    Corrected whole blood folate
    Glucose
Microbiological
    Oral rinse
    Swab of lesion
Mucosal biopsy

such as the floor of the mouth and the ventral surface of the tongue, demand careful consideration. More than one site may have to be biopsied.

At the time of initial biopsy any potential aetiological factors should be investigated and noted. This should include a record of tobacco and alcohol habits, microbiological investigations and haematological assessment (Table 8.2). Subsequent management of leukoplakia will depend on the findings of the initial biopsy. All possible aetiological factors must be eliminated and the histological appearance of the lesion reassessed after a period of 3 months. Haematological investigations are worthwhile in all such cases, as deficiency states lead to mucosal atrophy and, presumably, increased susceptibility to carcinogens.

Long-term review of all such cases is mandatory and not more than 2 years should elapse before further biopsy.

8.2 Squamous cell carcinoma

At the present time oral cancer accounts for only a small percentage (1–2%) of cancers occurring in the UK, but the number of new cases is rising, especially in females. In England and Wales it has been suggested that the number of deaths from oral cancer in females was 40% higher during the period 1980–84 when compared to that occurring between 1962–67. In addition it would appear that it is presenting at a younger age in males.

In 1990 there were approximately 2000 new cases of oral cancer and 1000 deaths from the disease in the UK. The incidence of the tumour increases with age, and the majority (85%) of cases occur in people over

Table 8.3 Survival from oral cancer (England and Wales 1981, from Cancer Research Campaign: Factsheet 14.3, 1990)

Site	Five-year survival (%)	
	Males	Females
Lip	94	71
Tongue	37	43
Gingivae	41	58
Floor of mouth	39	52
Other oral site	51	56

Table 8.4 Possible risk factors involved in the development of oral cancer

Tobacco
Alcohol
Nutritional deficiency
Candidal infection
Viral infection
Immunological factors

the age of 50 years. The disease is more common in men than women, but the ratio has fallen from approximately 5:1 in 1940 to 2:1 in 1990.

Overall, the 5-year survival from oral cancer is approximately 50%, although there are variations according to site (Table 8.3). Lip cancer has the best survival rate, possibly due to the increased likelihood of early detection and ease of treatment, whereas involvement of the floor of the mouth carries the worst prognosis. The extent or stage of the tumour is also a factor in the length of survival.

The clinical presentation of squamous cell carcinoma can vary greatly and range from a small erythematous patch of mucosa to a large area of ulceration or hyperplasia (Plates 18 and 19). The majority of squamous cell carcinomas develop in clinically normal mucosa, but may be preceded by a leukoplakia or erythroplakia. Unfortunately, oral cancer is painless in the early stages and therefore patients often present with advanced disease, including metastatic spread to regional lymph nodes.

A number of factors are associated with the development of oral cancer (Table 8.4), the two most important being tobacco and alcohol. In the UK, cigarette, cigar and pipe smoking account for most tobacco usage. Attempts to introduce smokeless chewing tobacco to the UK have met with opposition, and consumption is low. There is a direct

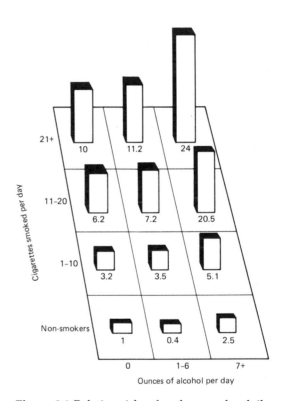

Figure 8.1 Relative risks of oral cancer by daily consumption of alcohol and cigarettes (males). (After McCoy, D. G. and Wynder, E. L. (1979) Etiology and preventive implications in alcohol carcinogenesis. *Cancer Research,* **39,** 2844–2850)

relationship between the number of cigarettes smoked per day and the risk of developing oral cancer (Figure 8.1). Moderate alcohol intake appears to reduce the risk of oral cancer, however excessive drinking is associated with a greater likelihood of occurrence of the disease. Interestingly, it is recognized that there is a synergistic effect between tobacco and alcohol, with a greatly increased risk if a patient has both habits rather than just one. Other factors, including diet, nutritional status, fungal infection, viral infection and iron deficiency have all been proposed as being important in the development of oral cancer.

Diagnosis

Squamous cell carcinoma *cannot* be diagnosed clinically and therefore histological examination of biopsy material from any suspected lesion is mandatory.

Treatment

In the UK treatment of oral cancer consists primarily of surgery and/or radiotherapy. Some patients may undergo surgery first, followed by a course of radiotherapy. Unfortunately, the postoperative survival of patients has changed little, due to death from new primary lesions or metastases.

Prevention

The obvious association between the development of oral cancer and the presence of habits of tobacco or alcohol consumption imply that elimination of these factors from the population should result in a substantial decrease in the development of the disease. All patients should be encouraged not to smoke and to limit their alcohol intake. If the outcome is influenced by early detection, then all health care workers should regularly undertake examination of the oral mucosa of their patients. Dental surgeons are ideally placed to carry out this examination and represent one of the key workers who could possibly improve the early detection of oral cancer. Any suspicious area of mucosa, such as a persistent area of ulceration, leukoplakia, or erythroplakia should be biopsied. This could be carried out in the general dental practice setting, but in cases of widespread mucosal involvement it may be more

sensible to refer the patient to a specialist oral medicine or oral surgery clinic.

8.3 Pigmented naevus and melanotic macule

Production of melanin by melanocytes within the oral mucosa produces pigmentation. The clinical appearance depends to some extent on the distribution and number of melanocytes and their activity. The term naevus is used to describe lesions where clusters of melanocytes occur. A number of types of naevi have been described, these include junctional naevus, compound naevus, intradermal naevus and blue naevus. Differentiation is important because the types behave differently with regard to progression to malignant melanoma.

The oral melanotic macule is a benign lesion which usually presents as a solitary area of brown pigmentation on the lower lip, gingivae or buccal mucosa.

Diagnosis

Diagnosis is based on the histological appearance of biopsy material.

Treatment

It has been suggested that all pigmented naevi should be surgically removed because all have potential to undergo malignant change. Clearly this is not always feasible when multiple lesions are present and therefore a decision has to be made on the basis of individual patients. All pigmental lesions should be kept under regular review.

8.4 Malignant melanoma

Although malignant melanoma, one of the deadliest of human neoplasms, accounts for 20% of skin cancer, it rarely occurs in the oral cavity. The aggressive behaviour and early metastatic spread of this tumour makes early diagnosis and treatment essential. An intra-oral malignant melanoma may develop in clinically normal mucosa, but frequently occurs within a pre-existing area of pigmentation. For this reason any area of mucosal pigmentation should be viewed seriously. Treatment of malignant melanoma is by radical surgical resection with removal of regional lymph nodes. Clinically, the pigmentation associated with a melanoma may range from light brown to dark blue/black.

Diagnosis

Diagnosis depends on the histological appearance of biopsy material.

Treatment

Treatment is based on radical surgical resection of the area of involvement, combined with regional lymph node dissection. The prognosis of this tumour is extremely poor with the 5-year survival rate in some studies being as low as 5%.

Further reading

Bryne, M. (1991) Prognostic value of various molecular and cellular features in oral squamous cell carcinomas: a review. *Journal of Oral Pathology and Medicine*, **20**, 413–420

Hogewind, W. F. C. and van der Waal, I. (1988) Leukoplakia of the labial commissure. *British Journal of Oral and Maxillofacial Surgery*, **26**, 133–140

Lamey, P-J. and Lewis, M. A. O. (1990) Oral medicine in practice; white patches. *British Dental Journal*, **168**, 147–152

McAndrew, P. G. (1990) Oral cancer and precancer: treatment. *British Dental Journal*, **168**, 191–198

Morton, M. and Roberts, H. (1990) Oral cancer and precancer: after-care and terminal care. *British Dental Journal*, **168**, 283–286

Pindborg, J. J. (1980) *Oral Cancer and Precancer*, Wright, Bristol

Scully, C. (1992) Oncogenes, onco-suppressors, carcinogenesis and oral cancer. *British Dental Journal*, **173**, 53–59

Shafer, W. G., Hine, M. K. and Levy, B. M. (1983) *A Textbook of Oral Pathology*, 4th ed. W. B. Saunders, Eastbourne

World Health Organization Collaborating Reference Centre for Oral Precancerous Lesions (1978) Definition of leukoplakia and related lesions. An aid to studies on oral precancer. *Oral Surgery, Oral Medicine, Oral Pathology*, **46**, 517–539

Part Four

Oral Manifestations of Systemic Disease

Chapter 9
Mucocutaneous disease

The oral mucosa has many structural similarities to that of the skin and, not surprisingly, a number of skin conditions may have oral manifestations. Mucocutaneous disorders may first present in the mouth, and early management may prevent subsequent cutaneous involvement.

9.1 Lichen planus

Lichen planus is a mucocutaneous disease which affects 0.5–2% of the population in the UK, with a slightly higher incidence in females than males. Approximately one-third of patients with oral lichen planus also have cutaneous lesions, but these usually resolve after 2–3 years, whereas oral lesions can persist for many years.

The oral manifestations of lichen planus consist of white patches or striae which may affect any site, often occurring in a symmetrical and bilateral distribution (Plate 20). The clinical appearance is variable and at least 6 forms have been described: reticular, papular, plaque-like, atrophic, erosive and (rare) bullous. However, clear division among the different types is often difficult and examination of the mucosa of an individual patient may reveal more than one subtype. In addition, the clinical signs and symptoms may change over a period of time. In view of this and the fact that the differentiation of type has little influence on clinical management, it is probably not necessary to subdivide lichen planus.

Cutaneous lesions of lichen planus, which usually present as pink papules, may develop at any site but occur most frequently on the flexor surfaces of the arms and legs. Fine white striae (Wickham's striae) may be seen on the surface of these papules.

Diagnosis

Although clinical diagnosis of oral lichen planus is helped by the presence of cutaneous lesions this should be confirmed by mucosal biopsy. The histological features include a well-defined band-like submucosal lymphocytic (T-cell) infiltrate, a feature which supports an autoimmune mechanism. It has also been suggested that Langerhan's cells play a role in the disease process. Choosing a representative area to biopsy may be difficult if involvement is widespread, and in this respect it has been suggested that tissue taken from the buccal mucosa is more likely to provide useful information than that from the tongue.

Treatment

Once the diagnosis has been confirmed histologically the patient should be reassured of the benign nature of the condition, especially if it is asymptomatic. It has been suggested that lichen planus, especially erosive lesions, may predispose to the development of oral cancer, but this view is by no means universally accepted. It would be wise, however, to maintain all patients with lichen planus on regular review and carry out further biopsies depending on the clinical progression.

In symptomatic cases the first line of treatment should consist of an antiseptic mouthwash, combined with topical steroid therapy in the form of either hydrocortisone hemisuccinate pellets (2.5 mg) or betamethasone sodium phosphate (0.5 mg) allowed to dissolve on the affected area 2–4 times daily. Other formats of topical steroid therapy, such as sprays, mouthwashes, creams and ointments, have been found to be beneficial for some patients. Intralesional injections of

triamcinolone have also been tried with variable success.

The possibility of a co-existing oral candidosis should be investigated and, if present, appropriate antifungal agents prescribed. Furthermore, stress appears to be an important precipitating factor, especially in older patients, and therefore anxiolytic therapy may be helpful.

In severe cases a short course of systemic steroid therapy may be required to alleviate acute symptoms. Griseofulvin, given systemically at a dose of 500 mg twice daily for 3 months, has been found to be helpful, although the mechanism by which a symptomatic improvement is achieved is not known. Baseline levels of liver enzymes should be determined prior to prescribing griseofulvin and following completion of the treatment. Patients taking an oral contraceptive should be advised that the efficacy of contraception is reduced by treatment with griseofulvin.

9.2 Lichenoid reaction

Lichenoid reactions are so named because of the similarity, both clinically and histologically, to lichen planus. Lesions can occur at any intraoral site, but in contrast to lichen planus it has been suggested that the distribution tends to be asymmetrical and involve the palate (Plate 21), although this has not as yet been proved by clinical studies. A wide range of drugs (antihypertensives, hypoglycaemics and non-steroidal anti-inflammatory agents), foodstuffs and dental materials (amalgam restorations) have been implicated in the development of mucosal lichenoid reactions.

Diagnosis

If lesions develop following the institution of drug therapy then there is likely to be a connection. Alternatively, if the lesions coincide with the presence of large old amalgams a sensitivity to mercury could be considered.

Mucosal biopsy is helpful in diagnosing a lichenoid reaction. In drug-induced lesions, a positive 'string of pearls' effect on indirect immunofluorescence would support a lichenoid reaction.

Treatment

If the patient is taking a medicine known to be associated with the occurrence of lichenoid reactions then consideration should be given to a change of therapy to a structurally unrelated drug with similar therapeutic effect. In the absence of obvious precipitating factors patch testing may be used to identify potential allergens, which can then be excluded.

9.3 Erythema multiforme

This self-limiting acute inflammatory condition is characterized by a variety of cutaneous lesions, including bullae, papules and macules. Skin involvement is classically described as concentric rings of erythema, the so-called 'target lesions'. The oral, ocular and genital mucosae may be affected, either alone or in combination with the skin. The orofacial lesions of erythema multiforme consist of blood-crusted lips and widespread painful oral ulceration (Plate 22).

The patient often has lymphadenopathy and feels generally unwell. The term 'Stevens-Johnson syndrome' has been used to describe severe cases with multiple site involvement. The symptoms of erythema multiforme usually resolve spontaneously within 10–14 days. However, patients can experience 2–3 recurrences of reduced severity within 2–3 years of the initial episode. The cause of erythema multiforme is uncertain but it has been associated with certain predisposing factors, including previous infection with *Herpes simplex* or *Mycoplasma pneumonia*, administration of systemic drugs, in particular sulphonamides and barbiturates, pregnancy, inflammatory bowel disease and exposure to sunlight.

Diagnosis

Diagnosis of erythema multiforme is usually made on clinical presentation and this is not difficult when skin lesions are also present. Primary herpetic gingivostomatitis, which like erythema multiforme is of rapid onset, is an important differential diagnosis to consider when involvement is limited to the oral mucosa.

Treatment

There is no specific treatment for erythema multiforme. If there is an association with recent drug therapy then this should be stopped. The provision of antiseptic mouthwash, and in severe cases a short course of systemic steroid therapy, has been found to be helpful; oral prednisolone is administered at a dose of 40 mg daily for 3–4 days, then gradually reduced over the following week. In severe cases hospitalization may be necessary to ensure adequate hydration. It is important to obtain an ophthalmic opinion for patients with eye involvement because blindness is a potential problem of severe erythema multiforme. Patients with recurrent disease should undergo patch testing to exclude hypersensitivity to foodstuffs, particularly the benzoate-based preservatives (E210–E219).

9.4 Pemphigoid

Pemphigoid is a relatively uncommon autoimmune vesiculobullous disease, which can affect the skin and oral mucosa. The condition is characterized by subepithelial bulla formation. Essentially there are two forms of pemphigoid and these are distinguished clinically by the site of involvement. In bullous pemphigoid, mucosal involvement is rare and cutaneous lesions predominate, whereas in mucous membrane pemphigoid (MMP) cutaneous involvement is rare. The oral presentation is variable but is often seen as areas of mucosal ulceration or desquamative gingivitis (Plate 23).

Diagnosis

Biopsy tissue, sent for histopathological analysis, should be examined for evidence of a submucosal split. Separate biopsy material should be sent on ice along with a 10 ml sample of clotted blood for immunofluorescence (IF) studies. Direct IF will show a linear deposition of IgG and usually C_3 along the basement membrane. Indirect IF is often negative.

Treatment

Steroids form the basis of treatment of pemphigoid, although there is a wide individual response to systemic or topical therapy. The majority of patients with MMP will respond to an initial course of systemic prednisolone followed by topical maintenance therapy. In some cases, however, it may be necessary to maintain systemic oral steroids with the addition of azathioprine. Dapsone has also been found to be effective in cases of MMP which do not respond to steroids. An ophthalmic opinion is required as the condition is associated with the development of conjunctival scarring.

9.5 Epidermolysis bullosa

Epidermolysis bullosa encompasses a group of uncommon conditions which are inherited in either an autosomal dominant or recessive pattern. All forms of the disease are characterized by fragility of the epithelium of the mouth or skin accompanied by bulla formation. The severity of the disease ranges from minor problems in the 'simple' and 'dystrophic' forms to severe involvement and possible death in the 'lethalis' form. Oral and perioral scar tissue can limit movement of the lips, tongue and mouth.

Diagnosis

Histopathological examination demonstrates features of subepithelial bullae. In one form of the disease there is true lysis of basal cells and electron microscopy can aid diagnosis.

Treatment

Systemic steroid therapy has been found to limit bulla formation. Phenytoin therapy may also be of some value, probably via an effect on fibroblast proliferation. Intraoral lesions can develop after minor trauma and therefore great care should be taken during any dental treatment.

9.6 Angina bullosa haemorrhagica

This blistering condition of the oral mucosa is characterized by the rapid appearance of a solitary blood-filled blister (haemorrhagic bulla), usually in the soft palate (Plate 24). Patients may complain of apparent tightness (angina) in the area immediately before and during the formation of swelling. The lesion invariably develops during eating and can be quite alarming to the patient, especially if haemorrhage occurs. In these circumstances, patients often seek immediate medical or dental attention. However, by the time of presentation the bulla may spontaneously discharge to leave an area of erosion. The cause of angina bullosa haemorrhagica is unknown, but it has been suggested that it could represent a mild localized form of epidermolysis bullosa. An association between the use of long-term steroid inhaler therapy and angina bullosa haemorrhagica has been described.

Diagnosis

Clinical history and appearance is often sufficient to make a diagnosis in an otherwise healthy patient. It is essential to exclude the presence of thrombocytopenia and therefore a full blood count should be undertaken.

Treatment

In the absence of any platelet deficiency the patient should be reassured and given an antiseptic mouthwash.

9.7 Pemphigus

Pemphigus comprises a group of vesiculo-bullous disorders characterized by involvement of the skin, mouth and other mucous membrane sites. Four main types are recognized: pemphigus vulgaris, pemphigus foliaceous, pemphigus erythematosis and pemphigus vegetans. Pemphigus arises because patients have a circulating immunoglobulin directed towards the desmosomal region of skin and mucous membranes. The antibody binding to these sites activates complement and plasminogen activator and subsequently acantholysis, vesicle formation, erosions and ulceration occur. The four types of pemphigus differ in the level of intraepithelial involvement in the disease; pemphigus vulgaris affects the whole epithelium and pemphigus foliaceous the upper prickle cell layer/spinous layer.

The clinical features of pemphigus are non-specific, with areas of erosion at any mucosal site, although non-keratinized sites appear to be affected most often. Skin lesions may or may not be present. Pemphigus is usually a disease of older people, with women being more affected than men. The oral mucosa is involved initially in about 50% of cases of pemphigus vulgaris (Plate 25) and indeed oral involvement can precede involvement at other sites. Because pemphigus is a life-threatening disease, it is important to confirm clinical suspicion of the disease by histological investigations at an early stage.

Diagnosis

Diagnosis is best confirmed by biopsy of an intact or recently ruptured bulla. Tissue should be sent for both routine histopathology and direct immunofluorescence. A blood sample should be sent for indirect immunofluorescence which will demonstrate circulating autoantibody (IgG). The titre of circulating antibody is important since it reflects the degree of disease activity.

Treatment

Once diagnosed it is best to arrange immediate hospital admission to allow drug therapy to be commenced and monitored. Pemphigus can rapidly involve large areas of skin and it is protein loss and electrolyte disturbance associated with this aspect of the disease which is responsible for mortality. The drug therapy of choice is systemic prednisolone, given at doses of up to 200 mg daily. Blood pressure needs careful monitoring in these early stages and antihypertensive drugs may be required. Once control is achieved and no new lesions develop and initial ones have healed, the dose of steroids is reduced to a maintenance level. Drugs such as azathioprine or cyclophosphamide have an important role in management as they allow the dose of steroid to be reduced. Since pemphigus is a lifelong disease, therapy cannot be discontinued. Complications of long-term steroid therapy, such as cataracts and duodenal ulcers, can occasionally develop and these need appropriate investigation and treatment.

9.8 Linear IgA disease

This rare disease is probably a variant of dermatitis herpetiformis. The disease produces persistent non-specific oral ulceration. Skin lesions also occur, particularly on the elbows, buttocks and scalp.

Diagnosis

Routine histopathological investigations show non-specific features, and therefore the diagnosis is made by demonstration of a linear deposition of IgA along the basement membrane using direct immunofluorescence.

Treatment

Systemic steroids or dapsone may produce clinical resolution of both the skin and oral lesions.

9.9 Dermatitis herpetiformis

Dermatitis herpetiformis is a rare chronic disease characterized by the development of crops of blisters on the skin or oral mucosa which may be preceded by erythematous patches. As the name implies, there is a clinical similarity to herpetic lesions. Oral lesions are occasionally the first manifestation of the condition. There is a relationship with coeliac disease and sensitivity to the α-gliadin fraction of wheat (gluten sensitivity).

Diagnosis

Histological features are non-specific, but direct immunofluorescence will reveal a granular deposition of IgA in the basement membrane zone.

Treatment

Treatment is based on the use of dapsone or sulphapyridine. Dietary avoidance of gluten can produce clinical resolution.

Further reading

Lewis, M. A. O., Lamey, P-J., Forsyth, A. and Gall, J. (1989) Recurrent erythema multiforme: a possible role of foodstuffs. *British Dental Journal*, **166**, 371–373

Mackie, R. M. (1986) *Clinical Dermatology*, 2nd edn, Oxford University Press, Oxford

Scully, C. and El-Kom, M. (1985). Lichen planus: review and update on pathogenesis. *Journal of Oral Pathology*, **14**, 431–458

Silverman, S. (1991) Lichen planus. *Current Opinion in Dentistry*, **1**, 769–772

Stephenson, P., Lamey P.-J., Scully, C., Prime, S. (1987) Angina bullosa haemorrhagica: clinical and laboratory features in 30 patients. *Oral Surgery, Oral Medicine, Oral Pathology*, **63**, 560–565

Walsh, L. J., Savage, N. W., Ishii, T. and Seymour, G. T. (1990) Immunopathogenesis of oral lichen planus. *Journal of Oral Pathology and Medicine*, **19**, 389–396

Williams, D. M. (1989) Vesiculo-bullous mucocutaneous disease: pemphigus vulgaris. *Journal of Oral Pathology and Medicine*, **18**, 544–553.

Williams, D. M. (1990) Vesiculo-bullous mucocutaneous disease: benign mucous membrane and bullous pemphigoid. *Journal of Oral Pathology and Medicine*, **19**, 16–23

Chapter 10
Gastrointestinal disease

The mouth forms the beginning of the gastrointestinal tract, and an abnormality of the oral mucosa can be an indication of the presence of lower tract disease. Oral lesions may either be part of a primary disease process occurring elsewhere in the gut or of a secondary manifestation of nutritional deficiency due to malabsorption or chronic blood loss.

10.1 Oesophageal reflux

Oesophageal reflux, possibly related to the presence of hiatus hernia, is one of the most common causes of dyspepsia. Patients will often complain of altered taste, especially in the morning, or of a burning sensation on the tongue. Regurgitation of gastric acid in these cases can lead to erosion of the palatal surfaces of the teeth, but in reality this is rarely a problem, except in the presence of pyloric stenosis.

Diagnosis

A barium meal examination in the Trendelenburg position can demonstrate oesophageal reflux and an associated hiatus hernia.

Treatment

The symptoms can be improved by adopting a diet of frequent small meals, the prescription of antacids and raising the head of the patient's bed.

10.2 Peptic ulceration

Peptic ulcers develop in the region of the acid secreting parts of the stomach (gastric ulcer) or duodenum (duodenal ulcer). Although there are no specific oral manifestations of peptic ulceration, chronic bleeding may produce recurrent oral ulceration, glossitis or cheilitis as a result of an associated iron deficiency anaemia.

Diagnosis

The medical diagnosis of peptic ulceration usually involves endoscopy or a barium meal examination.

Management

The mainstay of management involves H_2-receptor blocking drugs, such as cimetidine or ranitidine.

10.3 Crohn's disease

Crohn's disease is a granulomatous inflammatory disorder which may occur at any site along the gastrointestinal tract, but chiefly affects the terminal ileum. The onset of disease often occurs in the third decade, although there is also high peak incidence of initial presentation between the sixth and seventh decades. Oral lesions are common, with recurrent aphthous stomatitis occurring in approximately 20% of cases. Other oral manifestations include lip swelling, oedematous thickening of the buccal mucosa, mucosal tags, angular cheilitis and full width gingivitis (Plate 26). Pyostomatitis vegetans and epidermolysis bullosa acquisita may develop occasionally. Oral symptoms may precede any evidence of Crohn's disease within the lower gastrointestinal tract.

Diagnosis

Diagnosis is reached by demonstration of non-caseating epithelioid cell granulomata in biopsy material. Radiographic examination during barium enema should show ulceration and strictures. Clinically, perianal examination may reveal fistulae formation.

Treatment

Steroids, azathioprine and sulphonamides form the basis of systemic treatment. Any nutritional deficiency should be corrected.

10.4 Orofacial granulomatosis

The clinical signs of orofacial granulomatosis (OFG) are identical to those of Crohn's disease, and include lip swelling, angular cheilitis, oedematous thickening of the buccal mucosa, mucosal tags (particularly in the retromolar region), full width gingivitis and oral ulceration (Plate 27). Disease involvement is normally limited to the orofacial region. It is becoming increasingly apparent that OFG is likely to represent a hypersensitivity to foodstuffs, in particular benzoic acid, cinnamonaldehyde and chocolate.

Diagnosis

Histopathological examination of a mucosal biopsy should reveal non-caseating epithelioid cell granulomata. Patch testing using the Standard European Series will often identify potential allergens.

Treatment

In the short-term, use of the antihistamine agent terfenadine may be helpful in reducing the severity of any facial or lip swelling. Once an allergen has been identified the patient should be placed on an exclusion diet. Orofacial lesions will usually resolve within 3–18 months.

10.5 Ulcerative colitis

Ulcerative colitis is an inflammatory disease which affects the mucosa and submucosa of the colon and rectum. The onset is insidious, with a peak incidence in the third decade. Aphthous-like oral ulceration is the most common oral manifestation and occurs in between 4 and 20% of patients with ulcerative colitis. Other orofacial lesions associated with this condition include pyodema granulosum-like ulcers, pyostomatitis vegetans and erosive temporomandibular joint disease.

Diagnosis

Radiographic examination during barium enema should show loss of haustral pattern and shortening of the colon accompanied by ulceration and pseudopolyp formation.

Treatment

Treatment of ulcerative colitis is based on the use of sulphasalazine, a sulphonamide with anti-inflammatory properties, which has proven benefit in reducing the number and severity of relapses. In acute episodes systemic steroid therapy can be helpful.

10.6 Coeliac disease

In coeliac disease, subtotal villous atrophy occurs in the jejunum due to a reaction to the alpha gliadin component of wheat, rye or barley. The condition is relatively common, occurring in approximately 1:2000 individuals in the UK. Coeliac disease has been associated with histocompatibility antigens HLA-DR3 and HLA-D8. The presenting symptoms are variable, but can include oral ulceration secondary to a malabsorption.

Diagnosis

Diagnosis is by haematological screening to identify any nutritional deficiency, particularly of folic acid. Definitive diagnosis requires examination of a jejunal biopsy for evidence of villous atrophy.

Treatment

Once diagnosed the patient should be placed on a gluten-free diet and jejunal biopsy repeated after approximately 3 months. Oral ulcerative lesions normally respond to dietary exclusion, but folic acid supplementation may be required.

Further reading

Basu, M. K. and Asquith, P. (1980) Oral manifestations of inflammatory bowel disease. *Clinics in Gastroenterology*, **9**, 307–321

Basu, M. K. and Chesner, I. M. (1990) Diseases of the gastrointestinal tract. In *Oral Manifestations of Systemic Disease* (eds J. H. Jones and D. K. Mason), Baillière Tindall, London, pp. 783–799

Field, E. A. and Tyldesley, W. R. (1989) Oral Crohn's disease revisited – a 10-year review. *British Journal of Oral and Maxillofacial Surgery*, **27**, 114–123

Patton, D. W., Ferguson, M. M., Forsyth, A. and James, J. (1985) Orofacial granulomatosis: a possible allergic basis. *British Journal of Oral and Maxillofacial Surgery*, **23**, 235–242

Chapter 11
Haemopoetic disease and deficiency states

11.1 Anaemia	11.3 Amyloidosis
11.2 Leukaemia	

It has long been recognized that oral symptoms may be the first indication of the presence of an underlying haematological disorder or nutritional deficiency. The orofacial lesions seen most frequently in these circumstances are angular cheilitis, atrophic glossitis and oral ulceration.

11.1 Anaemia

Anaemia is defined as a reduced level of haemoglobin below that which is normal for the age and sex of the patient. It is usually associated in non-deficiency cases with a decreased number of erythrocytes. A patient may be termed anaemic when the concentration of haemoglobin falls below 12.5 g/dl in males and 12.0 g/dl in females. There are a number of causes of anaemia, including nutritional deficiency (iron, vitamin B_{12} or folic acid), reduced production of red cells (aplastic anaemia) and accelerated destruction of red cells (haemolytic anaemia).

Iron deficiency

Iron deficiency is not a disease in itself, but results from excessive loss, failure in utilization or, rarely, inadequate dietary intake. Most of the body's iron store is combined in haemoglobin within the red cells and a small amount is bound to the plasma protein transferrin. Iron deficiency is usually due to chronic blood loss, particularly as a result of menstrual bleeding in women. It has been estimated that approximately 8% of women of child-bearing age have deficiency anaemia, with a further 20% having iron deficiency (sideropenia).

Atrophic glossitis and angular cheilitis have been found to occur in approximately 40% and 15% of anaemic patients, respectively. The clinical presentation of the glossitis may range from a mild thinning of the papillae on the margins of the tongue to atrophy of the filiform and fungiform papillae in severe cases. There is also a generalized thinning of the oral mucosa, and patients may therefore be prone to the development of recurrent aphthous stomatitis.

Diagnosis

Haematological investigations should demonstrate a reduced level of ferritin or a low (<16%) ratio of serum iron to total iron binding capacity. Examination of blood film in an established case will reveal a reduced haemoglobin and red cell microcytosis.

Treatment

The underlying cause of iron deficiency should be identified prior to replacement therapy. A standard regime of iron therapy is ferrous sulphate in tablet form, 200 mg 8-hourly for 3 months. Oral symptoms usually respond quite rapidly to this form of treatment.

Kelly-Paterson (Plummer-Vinson) syndrome

This syndrome consists of iron deficiency anaemia, dysphagia and post-cricoid oesophageal stricture. Although uncommon, the syndrome is important because of an association with the development of post-cricoid and oral carcinoma.

Diagnosis

Diagnosis is based on clinical symptoms, findings of barium swallow and haematological evidence of iron deficiency.

Treatment

Iron deficiency should be eliminated by appropriate replacement therapy. Surgery may be required to correct the oesophageal defects.

Vitamin B_{12} deficiency

Inadequate dietary levels of vitamin B_{12} are extremely rare in developed countries, and

therefore vitamin B_{12} deficiency is usually a result of an absorption defect, such as pernicious anaemia or, less frequently, conditions affecting the terminal ileum, in particular Crohn's disease. A painful atrophic glossitis will develop in approximately half of patients with pernicious anaemia. Patients may also suffer from angular cheilitis or recurrent aphthous stomatitis.

Diagnosis

Haematological investigations will reveal a reduced level of vitamin B_{12} and, in established cases, red cell macrocytosis. The presence of autoantibodies to parietal cells and intrinsic factor should be determined in suspected cases of pernicious anaemia. The definitive diagnosis of pernicious anaemia requires a Schilling test.

Treatment

In pernicious anaemia, vitamin B_{12} supplements in the form of hydroxycobalamin given intramuscularly will be required for the remainder of the patient's life. The initial frequency of the administration will depend on the severity of the deficiency. Once adequate levels have been achieved a maintenance regime of 1000 μg every 2 months is usual. Oral lesions resolve rapidly following correction of the deficiency.

Folate deficiency

Deficiency of folate is often due to inadequate diet, but may occur as a result of malabsorption associated with the presence of a gastrointestinal abnormality, in particular coeliac disease. Folate deficiency is also a recognized side-effect of the use of phenytoin. Oral manifestations include glossitis, angular cheilitis and recurrent aphthous stomatitis.

Diagnosis

Haematological investigations will reveal a reduced level of corrected whole blood folate. A full blood count may reveal red cell macrocytosis in established deficiency. A jejunal biopsy is essential to exclude coeliac disease.

Treatment

If folate supplements are required then they can be given orally as a 5 mg tablet once daily. However, folic acid should be given with caution because there is a potential hazard of encouraging subacute combined degeneration of the spinal cord in patients who also have deficiency of vitamin B_{12}. Inappropriate supplement of folic acid may promote folate-dependent neoplasms, tumours and exacerbate epilepsy. Oral symptoms should respond following adequate replacement therapy.

Aplastic anaemia

This condition develops due to failure of the haemopoetic marrow, which leads to a pancytopenia with normochromic anaemia, granulocytopenia and thrombocytopenia. Opportunistic infections and haemorrhagic lesions of the oral mucosa and gingivae frequently develop.

Diagnosis

The most striking feature of a blood film in these patients is the marked paucity of all types of cells, in particular the red cell series.

Treatment

Management of aplastic anaemia is based on replacement therapy via transfusions. The anaemia may respond to steroid therapy, and marrow transplantation can be considered in some patients. Management of the oral lesions consists of minimizing the occurrence of opportunistic oral infections and maintaining adequate oral hygiene.

11.2 Leukaemia

Leukaemia is characterized by an abnormal and excessive proliferation of leukocyte precursors. The condition occurs in acute or chronic forms and may affect lymphocytes, monocytes and granulocytes. The acute forms are characterized by a rapidly progressive course with severe symptoms, including candidosis, gingival hypertrophy, petechiae, ulceration and herpetic infections (Plate 28). In contrast, progression in the chronic form is slow and oral manifestations are less severe.

Acute leukaemia

Acute lymphoblastic leukaemia (ALL) is the most common leukaemia of childhood, whilst acute myeloblastic leukaemia (AML) is the most common acute leukaemia of adulthood.

Diagnosis

Blood film investigation will determine which leucocyte population is involved. In addition, enzyme marker studies are of value in categorizing the individual form of leukaemia.

Treatment

Chemotherapy is the mainstay of treatment, but the role of bone marrow transplantation is becoming more widespread. Treatment of oral symptoms consists of minimizing opportunistic oral infections by the use of systemic or topical antiviral or antifungal agents. Maintenance of adequate oral hygiene can be helped by the regular use of chlorhexidine mouthwashes.

Chronic leukaemia

There are two main forms of chronic leukaemia, chronic lymphocytic (CLL) and chronic myeloid (CML). Although patients with chronic leukaemia may be asymptomatic, oral candidosis, herpetic infection, ulceration and petechiae can develop. As a generalization the lesions in the chronic leukaemia are less severe than those occurring in the acute forms of the disease.

Diagnosis

Blood film analysis confirms the identity of the predominant leucocyte precursor population.

Treatment

Treatment of chronic leukaemia involves radiotherapy, cytotoxic drugs or corticosteroids, depending on the individual case. Dental management is based on minimizing the occurrence of opportunistic mucosal infections and the maintenance of adequate oral hygiene.

11.3 Amyloidosis

Amyloidosis is characterized by the extracellular deposition of a group of proteins referred to as amyloid. The condition may occur in localized or systemic forms. The clinical presentation is extremely variable, ranging from an asymptomatic localized lesion to severe organ dysfunction as a result of widespread deposition of amyloid. The tongue is a common site of oral involvement.

Diagnosis

Staining of biopsy tissues with Congo red confirms the presence of amyloid.

Treatment

Localized deposits of amyloid can be removed surgically. There is no specific treatment for systemic amyloidosis, but treatment with steroids may be of value.

Further reading

Ferguson, M. M. (1990) Nutritional deficiency. In *Oral Manifestations of Systemic Disease* (eds J. H. Jones and D. K. Mason) Baillière Tindall, London, pp. 300–310

Ferguson, M. M., Dagg, J. H., Hunter, I. P. and Stephen, K. W. (1978) The presentation and management of oral lesions of leukaemia. *Journal of Dentistry*, **6**, 201–206

Maxymiw, W. G. and Wood, R. E. (1989) The role of dentistry in patients undergoing bone marrow transplantation. *British Dental Journal*, **167**, 229–234

Rennie, J. S., MacDonald, D. G. and Dagg, J. H. (1984) Iron and the oral epithelium: a review. *Journal of the Royal Society of Medicine*, **77**, 602–607

Scully C. and Gilmour, G. (1986) Neutropenia and dental patients. *British Dental Journal*, **160**, 43–46

Shepherd, J. P. (1978) The management of oral complications of leukaemia. *Oral Surgery, Oral Medicine, Oral Pathology*, **45**, 543–548

Wray, D. and Dagg, J. H. (1990) Diseases of the blood and blood-forming organs. In *Oral Manifestations of Systemic Disease*, (eds J. H. Jones and D. K. Mason) Baillière Tindall, London, pp. 660–713

Chapter 12
Immunological disease

Defence against microbial colonization is one of the main functions of the immune system, and therefore a defect in the system will result in the development of infections. This is well illustrated by the range of opportunistic infections which develop in the mouths of patients with AIDS. In addition to host defence, immune mechanisms are also involved in the mucosal autoimmune disorders pemphigus and pemphigoid (Chapter 9) and the systemic immune conditions rheumatoid arthritis and lupus erythematosus (Chapter 14).

12.1 HIV infection and AIDS

It is now accepted that the virus responsible for AIDS should be referred to as the human immunodeficiency virus (HIV). In the past this retrovirus was also known as lymphadenopathy virus (LAV) or human T-cell lymphotropic virus III (HTLV-III). HIV has the ability to attach to and kill CD4 lymphocytes, thereby reducing both cell-mediated and humoral immunity. The time from initial

exposure to the appearance of evidence of infection is variable and is generally accepted as ranging from 9 months to 2 years, although it is becoming apparent that it may be much longer than this. Incubation periods as short as 2 months or as long as 7 years have been reported.

Transmission of infection occurs via exchange of semen or blood during sexual intercourse, particularly between males, or passage of blood as a result of drug abuse habits. Maternal transmission of HIV also occurs *in utero*, producing paediatric AIDS. Prior to the recognition of AIDS, HIV was also spread as a result of the therapeutic transfusion of blood products. Screening of blood donors and heat-treatment of blood now prevents spread in this way.

At the beginning of 1992 anonymous screening of blood revealed that the evidence of exposure to HIV was detectable in approximately 1:1000 of the population in the UK, with much higher incidences in certain risk groups, such as homosexuals, prostitutes and intravenous drug abusers. Furthermore, it appears that its spread in the heterosexual community is increasing. The mortality from HIV infection approaches 100%, with more than 50% of patients with AIDS having already died.

The clinical features of HIV infection are variable and range from a 'glandular-fever' type syndrome following initial infection, to persistent generalized lymphadenopathy (PGL), an AIDS-related complex (ARC), and ultimately full-blown AIDS. In the late stage of infection the clinical symptoms are dominated by opportunistic infections, neurological disease and malignant neoplasms.

Diagnosis

Diagnosis of HIV infection is based on serological tests demonstrating exposure to the virus (see Chapter 4). The subsequent diagnosis of ARC or AIDS depends on the extent of the clinical symptoms and the severity of the immune deficiency.

Treatment

At the present time there is no specific treatment for HIV infection or AIDS. The antiviral agents zidovudine (azidothymidine, AZT) and acyclovir are used widely, but have met with limited success. Specific oral symptoms can be managed with appropriate antibiotics, antifungal agents or antiviral drugs.

Presentation and management of oral lesions of HIV infection

The spectrum of conditions associated with HIV infection is gradually evolving and oral or perioral lesions are frequently the presenting features. Unfortunately, the investigation of the oral manifestations has been complicated by lack of agreement on diagnostic criteria for individual lesions. It is hoped that an internationally accepted list of definitions and criteria will become available to allow multicentre studies in different countries of the world to become possible. The conditions seen most frequently in HIV are

Table 12.1 Oral manifestations of HIV infection

Common lesions
  Candidosis
    Pseudomembranous
    Erythematous
    Hyperplastic
    Angular cheilitis
  Gingivitis/periodontitis
    'HIV associated' gingivitis
    'HIV associated' periodontitis
    Necrotizing periodontitis
    Necrotizing stomatitis
  Herpes simplex
    Intraoral lesions
    Perioral lesions
  Varicella zoster
    Herpes zoster
  Hairy leukoplakia
  Kaposi's sarcoma

Rare lesions
  Salivary gland disease
  Recurrent aphthous stomatitis
  Human papilloma virus
  Lymphoma
  Neuropathies
  Hyperpigmentation
  Lichenoid drug reactions

listed in Table 12.1, and these will be discussed below.

Candidosis

Oral candidosis is often the initial symptom of HIV infection and exists in four distinct forms; pseudomembranous, erythematous (atrophic), hyperplastic and angular cheilitis. Levels of *Candida albicans* in saliva are increased in HIV-positive individuals and appear to rise with a reduction in the CD4:CD8 lymphocyte ratio.

The pseudomembranous form presents as semi-adherent white/yellow membranes which can be removed with a swab to reveal an erythematous underlying mucosa. Any area of the mucosa may be affected, but the tongue and soft palate are most frequently involved. The condition is usually acute, but in HIV-infected patients it may persist for several months. The erythematous forms of candidosis is characteristically seen as a red area of depapillation on the dorsum of the tongue. Chronic hyperplastic candidosis in HIV is the rarest subtype but may produce adherent white patches affecting both buccal mucosae. It is important to distinguish chronic hyperplastic candidosis from hairy leukoplakia, which often also contains candida on its surface. Angular cheilitis, consisting of painful red fissures at the angles of the mouth, may accompany any form of candidosis, especially if the patient is HIV-positive.

Management of oral candidosis in HIV infection consists of the use of topical agents, such as nystatin or amphotericin, but these are sometimes ineffective and relapses are common. It is often necessary therefore to provide systemic therapy in the form of ketoconazole, fluconazole or itraconazole. The use of these systemic agents has been very effective, but there is concern about the emergence of resistance among strains of candida.

Gingivitis/periodontitis

The health of the gingivae and periodontum can deteriorate rapidly in HIV-positive patients. The severity and pattern of periodontal disease in these individuals has led to the use of the terms 'HIV associated gingivitis' and 'HIV associated periodontitis'. However, at the present time there is still uncertainty about the exact terminology and criteria for the types of periodontal lesions seen. There would certainly appear to be adequate evidence to support the fact that HIV patients do suffer from a form of rapidly destructive disease which has been termed necrotizing periodontitis. Further study of the periodontal involvement in HIV is required to establish uniformly accepted definitions and criteria.

Management of periodontal lesions in HIV should consist of the provision of professional local hygiene measures combined with patient oral hygiene involving the use of chlorhexidine mouthwashes. Metronida-

zole is helpful in alleviating symptoms of necrotizing periodontitis.

Herpes simplex

Herpes simplex virus infection is relatively common in HIV and can present either periorally as herpes labialis or intraorally as areas of ulceration. Symptoms are particularly severe and prolonged. Acyclovir (200 mg orally five times daily), is the mainstay of treatment and is extremely effective both at treating established lesions and suppressing recurrences. *Herpes simplex* resistance to acyclovir has been reported and if this occurs the use of intravenous foscarnet (50 mg/kg/day) has been suggested.

Varicella zoster

Reactivation of *Varicella zoster* virus can sometimes produce intraoral and cutaneous herpes zoster in HIV patients. Management of this condition consists of the use of acyclovir (800 mg orally five times daily).

Hairy leukoplakia

Hairy leukoplakia was pathognomonic of HIV infection, but recently the lesion has been described in other severely immunocompromised patients. The classical appearance of hairy leukoplakia is a painless corrugated 'hairy' white patch affecting the lateral borders of the tongue (Plate 29). Biopsy will reveal characteristic histological features of hyperparakeratosis with surface projections, hyperplasia of the prickle cell layer, koilocytes, candidal hyphae and scanty inflammatory cell infiltrate. Special investigations will reveal the presence of Epstein-Barr virus. Although hairy leukoplakia is usually seen on the tongue, it has also been described as affecting the gingivae and buccal mucosa. Development of hairy leukoplakia is regarded at the present time as an indicator of poor prognosis.

Treatment of hairy leukoplakia depends on individual cases and the extent of involvement since the condition is usually asymptomatic. Lesions will regress in response to acyclovir but are likely to return once therapy has been discontinued.

Kaposi's sarcoma

Oral Kaposi's sarcoma is a malignant endothelial cell tumour which develops almost exclusively in HIV positive patients. Most lesions arise in the palate and present as a blood/purple patch in the early stage (Plate 30) which become more exophytic as the condition develops. A possible role of cytomegalovirus in Kaposi's sarcoma has been suggested, but this has not yet been proved.

Treatment options consist of local excision, intralesional vinblastine or radiotherapy depending on the site and extent of the sarcoma.

Miscellaneous rare lesions

Swelling of the major salivary glands has been described in HIV patients and sialographic examination may reveal sialectasis similar to that seen in Sjögren's syndrome. A reduction in salivary flow rates is well recognized and therefore the patients may suffer from the effects of xerostomia. Management in this situation is as for other causes of xerostomia and involves preventive dental measures and the provision of artificial saliva substitutes.

Ulcers identical to each of the three types of recurrent aphthous stomatitis may develop at the time of HIV sero-conversion and subsequently cause troublesome symptoms. Microbiological and histological investigations should be undertaken if aphthae-like lesions persist, in order to exclude other causes of oral ulceration. Treatment is based on the use of topical steroids and this is effective in the majority of patients. Occasionally systemic steroid or thalidomide might be the only effective therapy.

Human papilloma virus types 7, 13, 18 and 32 have been implicated in the development of oral papillomatous conditions in HIV infection. Treatment of these conditions is by excision or cryotherapy as necessary. HIV infection is also associated with an increased incidence of non-Hodgkin's lymphoma which can be managed by radiotherapy. Neurological changes involving palsy of the facial nerve and paraesthesia/anaesthesia of the trigeminal nerve have been described in HIV-positive individuals. A brown-black hyperpigmentation of the oral mucosa may also develop in patients with HIV, and it has been suggested in some patients that this may be in part due to a side-effect of zidovudine.

12.2 Myasthenia gravis

This autoimmune condition usually affects women below the age of 35 years. The onset of disease is insidious and presents as muscle weakness. Ptosis, loss of facial expression, and difficulty with speech, chewing or swallowing, can be prominent features when the orofacial musculature is involved.

Diagnosis

Patients with myasthenia gravis have a demonstrable circulating autoantibody directed towards the nicotinic receptors of striated muscles. Electromyography will also be abnormal.

Treatment

Patients with this condition should be referred to a neurologist. Effective treatment involves the use of anticholinesterases.

12.3 Pernicious anaemia

This autoimmune disease usually presents in the middle-aged or elderly woman. Patients do not have specific gastrointestinal problems but will suffer symptoms due to the resultant vitamin B_{12} deficiency. The oral presentation can involve glossitis, angular cheilitis, burning mouth syndrome or recurrent oral ulceration.

Diagnosis

The basis of the pernicious anaemia is reduced availability of intrinsic factor in the stomach due to the presence of autoantibodies towards the parietal cells and intrinsic factor itself. Demonstration of these autoantibodies strongly suggest a diagnosis of pernicious anaemia. A Schilling test is used to confirm the diagnosis.

Treatment

Treatment requires lifelong vitamin B_{12} replacement in the form of hydroxocobalamin, given intramuscularly.

Further reading

Farthing, C. F., Brown, S. E., Staughton, R. C. D., Cream, J. J. and Muhlemann, M. (1986) *A Colour Atlas of AIDS*, Wolfe Medical Publications, London

Greenspan, D., Greenspan, J. S., Schiodt, M. and Pindborg, J. J. (1990) *Aids and the Mouth*, Munksgaard, Copenhagen

Greenspan, J. S., Barr, C. E., Sciubba, J. J. and Winkler, J. R. (1992) Oral manifestation of HIV infection: definition, diagnostic criteria and principles of therapy. *Oral Surgery, Oral Medicine, Oral Pathology*, **73**, 142–144

Lehner, T. (1992) *Immunology of Oral Diseases*, Blackwell Scientific Publications, Oxford

Peterson, D. E., Greenspan, D. and Squirer, C. A. (1992) Oral infections in the immunocompromised host. *Journal of Oral Pathology and Medicine*, **21**, 193–198

Reichart, P. A. (1991) Oral manifestations of recently described viral infections, including AIDS. *Current Opinion in Dentistry*, **1**, 377–383

Samaranayake, L. P. and Holmstrup, P. (1989) Oral candidiasis and human immunodeficiency virus infection. *Journal of Oral Pathology and Medicine*, **18**, 554–564

Scully, C. and McCarthy, G. (1992) Management of oral health in person with HIV infection. *Oral Surgery, Oral Medicine, Oral Pathology*, **73**, 215–225

Smith, A. J. and Walker, D. M. (1992) The origins of the human immunodeficiency viruses: an update. *Journal of Oral Pathology and Medicine*, **21**, 145–149

Chapter 13
Endocrine disease

13.1 Acromegaly

13.2 Addison's disease

13.3 Cushing's disease

13.4 Diabetes mellitus

13.5 Hypothyroidism

13.6 Hyperthyroidism

13.7 Hyperparathyroidism

13.8 Puberty, pregnancy and climacteric

The endocrine system consists of a number of ductless glands which secrete specific hormones that regulate cellular metabolism. Complex inter-relationships exist between these hormones and therefore altered secretion by one gland often produces changes in other glands. Endocrine dysfunction may cause oral symptoms either as a direct hormonal effect or as a result of associated secondary changes. In general, specific mucosal lesions due to endocrine abnormalities are rare and those which are seen are often associated with changes occurring in normal life (puberty, pregnancy and menopause).

13.1 Acromegaly

A number of hormones are secreted by the pituitary gland, but only somatotropin (growth hormone) has a direct effect on the oral tissues. The oral symptoms produced by excessive secretion of somatotropin will depend on the age of the patient and whether bone growth centres are still active. Hypersecretion during childhood will result in gigantism, whilst in adulthood it will produce acromegaly. Orofacial manifestations of acromegaly include mandibular prognathism, spacing of the teeth, malocclusion and enlargement of the salivary glands.

Diagnosis

Haematological investigation should detect elevated levels of growth hormone. A lateral skull radiograph may reveal evidence of pituitary enlargement.

Treatment

Treatment is by surgical resection of the underlying pituitary adenoma.

13.2 Addison's disease

Addison's disease is characterized by reduced secretion of glucocorticoids and mineralocorticoids. The disease is rare but may occur either as a result of hyposecretion of adrenocorticotrophic hormone (ACTH) by the pituitary gland or destruction of the adrenal cortex. Addison's disease is often caused by an autoimmune disorder in which autoantibodies to the adrenal cortex are produced. Features of Addison's disease include fatigue, lethargy, weight loss, nausea and hyperpigmentation of the skin. Pigmentation of the oral mucosa also occurs in approximately three-quarters of patients. More recently Addison's disease has been associated with HIV infection.

Diagnosis

The patient will usually be hypotensive. Serological investigation may reveal a reduced level of sodium along with raised potassium. Adrenal function can be assessed by noting the response to synthetic ACTH (Synacthen test).

Treatment

Glucocorticoids and mineralcorticoids given systemically will correct any deficiencies.

13.3 Cushing's disease

Cushing's disease is a rare disorder caused by excessive production of glucocorticoids due to hypersecretion of ACTH by a pituitary adenoma or the presence of an adenoma of the adrenal cortex. A clinically similar but far more common condition is Cushing's syndrome, which may be caused by primary adrenal disease or more frequently by the therapeutic administration of systemic corticosteroid therapy. The clinical features of Cushing's syndrome include weight gain, particularly on the face (moon face) and back (buffalo hump), diabetes, acne, psychosis and hirsutism.

Diagnosis

Diagnosis is based on the detection of elevated levels of plasma cortisol (Cushing's disease) or a history of corticosteroid treatment (Cushing's syndrome).

Treatment

The treatment is by surgical resection of any pituitary or adrenal tumour. In Cushing's syndrome consideration should be given to substituting corticosteroid therapy with alternative non-steroidal agents.

13.4 Diabetes mellitus

Diabetes mellitus occurs as a result of an absolute or relative deficiency of insulin, which is produced by the islet cells of the pancreas. Two types of the disease exist: type I (insulin-dependent diabetes) which usually presents in childhood and type II (non-insulin-dependent diabetes) which develops primarily in adulthood. Some degree of diabetes is probably present in approximately 2% of the adult population in the UK but it is only recognized in about half of these individuals. The onset of type I diabetes is usually acute, consisting of polyuria, thirst and weight loss, whilst the onset of type II diabetes is more protracted. In adequately controlled sufferers there should be no oral manifestations, but a range of symptoms may be present prior to diagnosis and in known diabetics with poor glycaemic control.

Oral signs and symptoms include dry mouth, candidosis, periodontal disease, sialosis and burning mouth syndrome. Diabetic patients may also develop lichenoid reactions of the oral mucosa as a result of their oral hypoglycaemic agents.

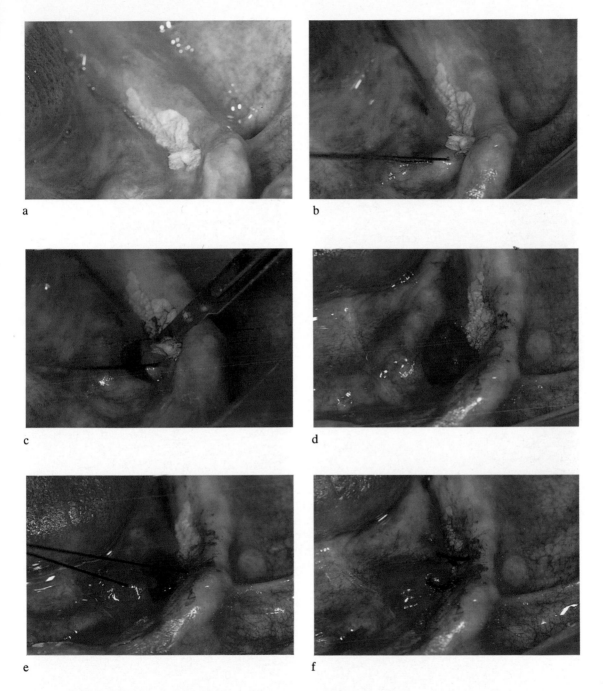

Plates 1 a–f Stages of mucosal biopsy. (a) Lesion in the lower left premolar region. (b) Suture placed within normal tissue anterior to the area to be biopsied. (c) Lower and upper incisions are made to form an elipse of tissue. (d) Defect created by biopsy. (e) Wound closed using interrupted black silk sutures. (f) Primary closure achieved.

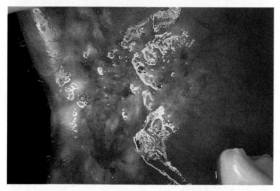

Plate 2 Acute pseudomembraneous candidosis

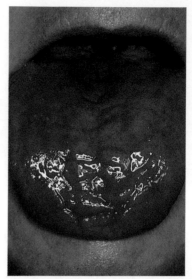

Plate 3 Acute erythematous candidosis

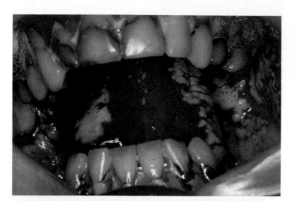

Plate 4 Chronic hyperplastic candidosis

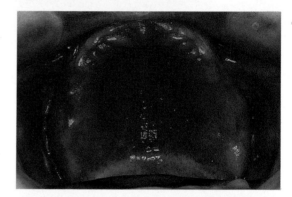

Plate 5 Chronic erythematous candidosis

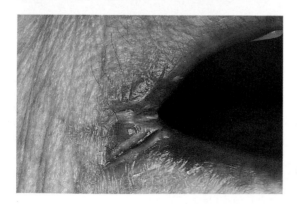

Plate 6 Angular cheilitis

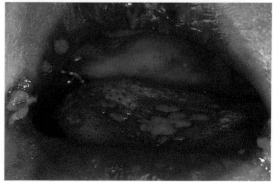

Plate 7 Acute primary herpetic gingivostomatitis

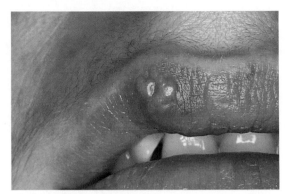

Plate 8 Herpes labialis

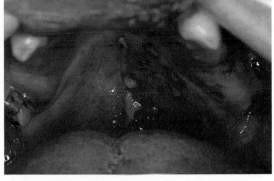

Plate 9 Herpes zoster

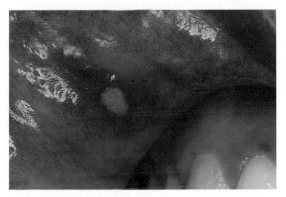

Plate 10 Minor aphthous stomatitis

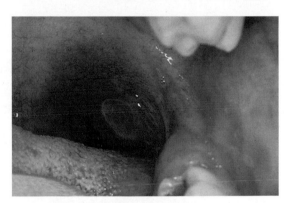

Plate 11 Major aphthous stomatitis

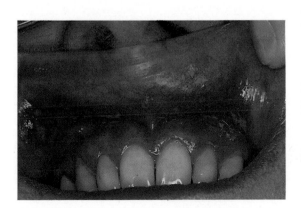

Plate 12 Herpetiform aphthous stomatitis

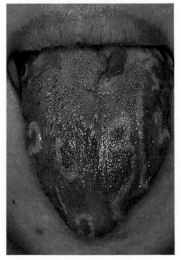

Plate 13 Geographic tongue

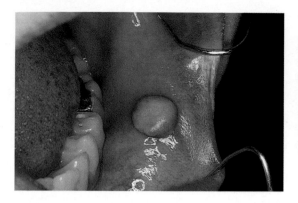

Plate 14 Fibroepithelial polyp

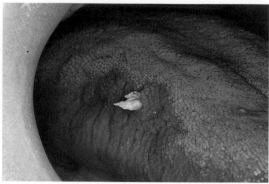

Plate 15 Squamous cell papilloma

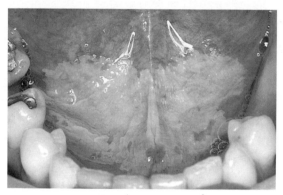

Plate 16 Leukoplakia /Sublingual Keratosis

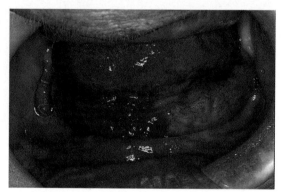

Plate 17 Erythroplakia

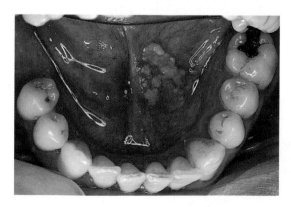

Plate 18 Early squamous cell carcinoma

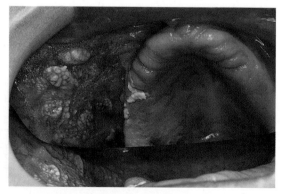

Plate 19 Late stage carcinoma

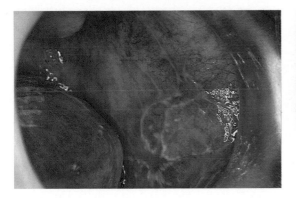

Plate 20 Lichen planus

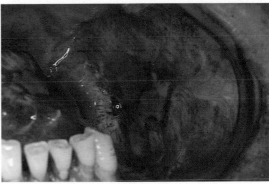

Plate 21 Lichenoid reaction

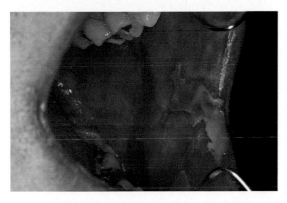

Plate 22 Erythema multiforme

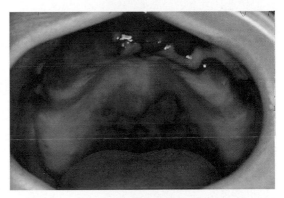

Plate 23 Benign mucous membrane pemphigoid

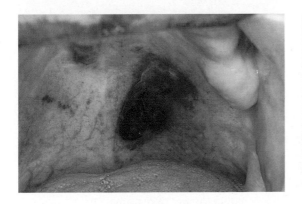

Plate 24 Angina bullosa haemorrhagica

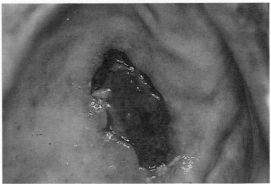

Plate 25 Pemphigus

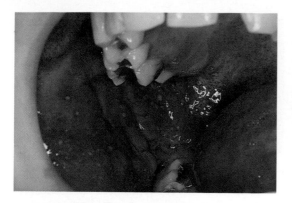

Plate 26 Crohn's disease

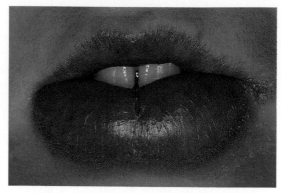

Plate 27 Orofacial granulomatosis

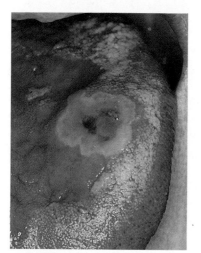

Plate 28 Leukaemia

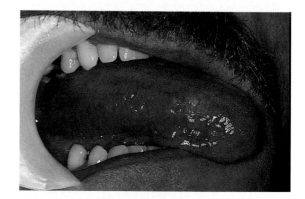

Plate 29 HIV – hairy leukoplakia

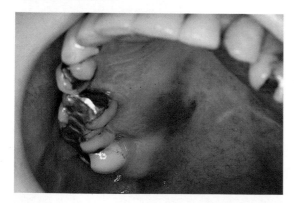

Plate 30 HIV – Kaposi's sarcoma

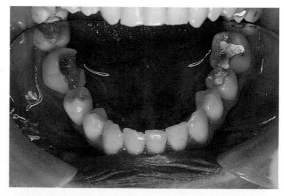

Plate 31 Schizophrenic patient who presented after removing many of her amalgam restorations

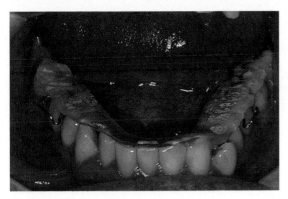

Plate 32 Acrylic splint *in situ*

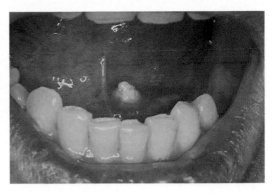

Plate 33 Salivary calculus at the submandibular duct orifice

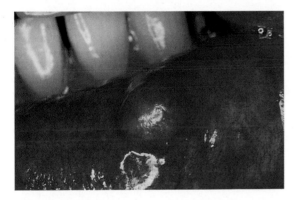

Plate 34 Mucocele arising beneath the lower labial mucosa

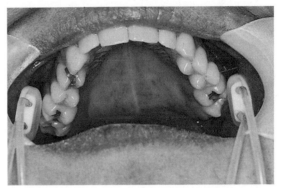

Plate 35 Carlsson Crittenden cup over parotid orifice

Diagnosis

Diagnosis is based on the detection of elevated levels of glucose in the blood or urine. Chairside tests which give an indication of levels of glucose are available and easy to use but are not suffiently accurate for diagnostic purposes. Chemical assessment of venous plasma glucose level is the most accurate assay. The degree or severity of diabetes can be assessed by a glucose tolerance test. A serum glucose level of over 11 mmol/l 2 hours after a 75 g glucose load is diagnostic of diabetes mellitus.

Treatment

Treatment is by maintenance of adequate blood glucose levels, by dietary control and/or oral hypoglycaemic agents/insulin injections.

13.5 Hypothyroidism

A number of orofacial signs and symptoms can be produced as a result of insufficient secretion of thyroxine and tri-iodothyronine by the thyroid gland. If such a problem occurs in young children the characteristic appearance of cretinism occurs. The orofacial features of cretinism include enlarged lips, macroglossia, an underdeveloped mandible and maxillary hypoplasia. In adults, hypothyroidism produces a puffy, myxodematous appearance of the face with loss of the eyebrows.

Diagnosis

Diagnosis is made haematologically by detection of a reduced free thyroxine index. Thyroid stimulating hormone (TSH) is raised in primary hypothyroidism but depressed in secondary hypothyroidism.

Treatment

Treatment consists of thyroxine supplements given orally.

13.6 Hyperthyroidism

Excessive secretion of thyroid hormones causes weight loss, anaemia, vomiting, anxiety and sweating. The classical oro-facial signs involve the eyes and consist of lid lag, lid retraction and exophthalmos.

Diagnosis

Diagnosis is made chemically by detection of altered levels of tri-iodothyronine, thyroxine and free thyroxine index.

Treatment

Treatment may be medical or surgical. Xerostomia has been reported following the use of radioactive iodine therapy.

13.7 Hyperparathyroidism

Primary hyperparathyroidism is caused by an adenoma of one or more of the parathyroid glands, whereas secondary hyperparathyroidism is usually secondary to renal disease. A specific giant cell lesion termed a brown tumour or osteitis fibrosis cystica may develop intraorally in patients with hyperparathyroidism. Alteration in levels of parathormone affect bone turnover and radiographic examination may reveal complete or partial loss of the lamina dura with a ground-glass appearance of the alveolar bone.

Diagnosis

Chemical investigation will reveal an elevated serum calcium and increased level of alkaline phosphatase (see Table 15.1). Isoenzyme studies will show the alkaline phosphatase to be of bony origin.

Treatment

Treatment is by surgical removal of the parathyroid glands and provision of vitamin D therapy. Oral lesions should resolve fully following adequate treatment of the underlying systemic disorder.

13.8 Puberty, pregnancy and climacteric

Alterations of sex hormone levels may produce a number of oral changes, particularly in females. At the time of puberty children of either sex may develop a gingivitis accompanied by swelling of the interdental papillae. A pronounced gingival lesion, often referred to as pregnancy epulis, can develop during pregnancy.

The development of recurrent aphthous stomatitis during the luteal phase of the menstrual cycle and absence of ulceration during pregnancy has been described in some women. At the present time the exact relationship between sex hormones and the development of aphthae is not clear.

Burning mouth syndrome has been attributable to the hormonal changes occurring in menopausal women.

Further reading

Basker, R. M., Sturdee, D. W. and Davenport, J. C. (1978) Patients with burning mouths. *British Dental Journal*, **145**, 9–16

Ferguson, M. M., and Silverman, S. (1990) Endocrine Disorders. In *Oral Manifestations of Systemic Disease* (eds J. H. Jones and D. K. Mason), Baillière Tindall, London, pp. 593–615

Ferguson, M. M., Hart, D. McK., Lindsay, R. and Stephen, K. W. (1978) Progestogen therapy for menstrually related aphthae. *International Journal of Oral Surgery* **7**, 463–470

Gibson, J., Lamey, P-J., Lewis, M. A. O. and Frier, B. M. (1990) Oral manifestations of previously undiagnosed non-insulin dependent diabetes mellitus. *Journal of Oral Pathology and Medicine* **19**, 284–287

Lamey, P-J. and Lamb, A. B. (1988) Prospective study of the aetiological factors in burning mouth syndrome. *British Dental Journal* **296**, 1243–1246

Lamey, P-J. Carmichael, F. A. and Scully, C. (1985) Oral pigmentation, Addison's disease and the results of screening for adrenocortical insufficiency. *British Dental Journal* **158**, 297–298

MacDonald, D. G., and Boyle, I. T. Skeletal diseases. In *Oral Manifestations of Systemic Disease* (eds J. H. Jones and D. K. Mason), Baillière Tindall, London, pp. 616–659

Chapter 14
Connective tissue disease

<table>
<tr><td>14.1 Rheumatoid arthritis</td><td>14.3 Progressive systemic sclerosis (scleroderma)</td></tr>
<tr><td>14.2 Lupus erythematosus</td><td>14.4 Reiter's syndrome</td></tr>
</table>

There is a group of conditions including rheumatoid arthritis, systemic lupus erythematosus and progressive systemic sclerosis, that are collectively known as the 'connective tissue diseases'. The cause of these disorders is unknown, but it is likely to involve an altered host immunological response. The term 'connective tissue disease' only indicates the principal tissue involved and each condition may have a range of oral manifestations.

14.1 Rheumatoid arthritis

This multisystem disease affects 2% of the UK population, with a peak onset in the fourth decade and a higher incidence in women. The onset of symptoms is usually insidious and first affects the small joints of the hands or feet. The metacarpophalangeal and proximal interphalangeal joints become progressively painful and swollen, leading to limitation of movement, which may then spread to the wrists, elbows and knees (Figure 14.1).

Rheumatoid arthritis may be the connective tissue component of Sjögren's syndrome, and sufferers may therefore complain of xerostomia. A minority (10–15%) of patients with rheumatoid arthritis complain of limitation and stiffness of the temporomandibular joints, although pain is not usually a feature. The anti-inflammatory drugs used to treat rheumatoid arthritis have been implicated in the occurrence of

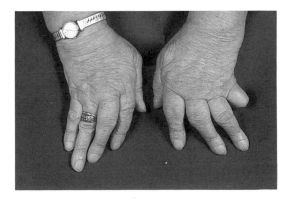

Figure 14.1 Rheumatoid arthritis

lichenoid reactions. Rheumatoid arthritis is associated with iron deficiency anaemia, and patients may therefore suffer from glossitis, angular cheilitis or recurrent aphthous stomatitis.

Diagnosis

Rheumatoid factor, an autoantibody against the patient's own immunoglobulins, is positive in approximately 75% of patients with rheumatoid arthritis (RA latex test). The Rose-Waaler test is less sensitive, but more specific for rheumatoid arthritis.

Treatment

Treatment depends on the severity of the disease, but is likely to involve the use of aspirin, anti-inflammatory agents, gold, steroids and/or physiotherapy. Treatment of all the oral manifestations are usually based on the relief of xerostomia (see Chapter 6). Limitations of the patient's dexterity may complicate the maintenance of adequate oral hygiene.

14.2 Lupus erythematosus

Lupus erythematosus is an example of a 'typical' autoimmune disease which has a wide variation of clinical features. There are two main clinical divisions of the conditions, namely discoid lupus erythematosus (DLE) and systemic lupus erythematosus (SLE) which may represent different ends of the spectrum of disease activity. In DLE involvement is restricted and patients predominantly complain of cutaneous lesions. Skin lesions, in particular an erythematous rash over the malar region and bridge of the nose (butterfly rash), occur in SLE, but systemic involvement, such as nephritis and anaemia, is also present. The oral manifestations of DLE and SLE are indistinguishable and consist of atrophic areas of mucosa with peripheral erythema and white striae. The buccal and labial mucosae are often involved, usually bilaterally. Approximately 30% of patients with SLE will suffer xerostomia as part of Sjögren's syndrome.

Diagnosis

The publication of the diagnostic and therapeutic criteria by the American Rheumatism Association has aided diagnosis of SLE since the disease may involve almost any body system. Oral ulceration is listed as a major diagnostic feature of SLE and biopsy of oral lesions can be helpful. Serological diagnosis is based on detection of autoantibodies against double-stranded DNA.

Treatment

Corticosteroids are the mainstay of drug therapy, but other drugs such as chloroquine may also be effective.

14.3 Progressive systemic sclerosis (scleroderma)

This condition is characterized by a chronic diffuse sclerosis of the skin, gastrointestinal tract, heart, lungs and kidneys. Clinical symptoms will depend on the extent of involvement. However, when the skin of the face is involved the patient's face may develop a pinched appearance and the lips may become drawn causing limited mouth opening. Progressive systemic sclerosis may be the connective tissue component of Sjögren's syndrome and patients may therefore often complain of xerostomia. CREST syndrome, consisting of Calcinosis, Raynaud's phenomenon, oEsophageal stricture, Sclerodactyly and Telangectasia is related to progressive systemic sclerosis.

Diagnosis

A raised erythrocyte sedimentation rate and hypergammaglobulinaemia are usually present. Antinuclear antibody is present in approximately 70% of patients.

Treatment

No specific treatment is available, although penicillamine may be used. Corticosteroids are contraindicated in most cases. Oral aspects of management include the elimination of complications related to xerostomia.

14.4 Reiter's syndrome

Reiter's syndrome consists of arthritis, urethritis and conjunctivitis and occurs mainly in men between 20 and 35 years of age. The cause of Reiter's syndrome may be based on a postinfective response, since cases are known to follow a sexually transmitted disease. At the present time the exact nature of the condition is uncertain. Oral lesions, consisting of painful superficial ulceration, particularly of the tongue, buccal mucosa and palate, are a frequent feature.

Diagnosis

Clinical diagnosis would be supported by detection of a raised erythrocyte sedimenta-tion rate. The condition is associated with HLA-B27.

Treatment

Anti-inflammatory drugs have been tried with variable success. No specific treatment is required for the oral involvement.

Further reading

Greenspan, J. S. and Daniels, T. E. (1990) Connective tissue and granulomatosus diseases of doubtful origin. In *Oral Manifestations of Systemic Disease* (eds J. H. Jones and D. K. Mason), Baillière Tindall, London, pp. 271–299

Maustein, U. F., Hermann, K. and Böhme, H. J. (1986) Pathogenesis of progressive systemic sclerosis. *International Journal of Dermatology* **25**, 286–293

Pindborg J. J. (1990) Diseases of the skin. In *Oral Manifestations of Systemic Disease* (eds J. H. Jones and D. K. Mason), Baillière Tindall, London, pp. 537–592

Schiødt, M. (1984) Oral manifestations of lupus erythematous. *International Journal of Oral Surgery*, **13**, 101–147

Chapter 15
Skeletal disease

| 15.1 Fibrous dysplasia | 15.2 Paget's disease (osteitis deformans) |

A number of bone disorders with either a congenital, metabolic or inflammatory basis, may affect the orofacial region. Most of these are rare, although Paget's disease and fibrous dysplasia do occur relatively commonly. Diagnosis of bone disorders usually involves chemical examination of serum levels of calcium, phosphate and alkaline phosphatase and radiological examination of affected tissues.

15.1 Fibrous dysplasia

Fibrous dysplasia occurs in two forms, monostotic, in which a single bone is affected, and polyostotic, in which there is involvement at multiple sites. The cause of the condition is unknown, but it is best regarded as a developmental disorder in which bone is replaced by fibrous tissue. Fibrous dysplasia involving in the jaws usually represents a monostotic form of the disorder. The maxilla is affected more frequently than the mandible. Clinical presentation is characterized by the development of a painless and slowly progressive unilateral swelling during childhood. The jaws are involved in approximately 20% of cases of polyostotic fibrous dysplasia. Approximately half of the patients with the polyostotic form of the condition will also have skin pigmentation. The presence of fibrous dysplasia combined with pigmentation and precocious puberty in females is referred to as Albright's syndrome.

Diagnosis

Chemical investigation will reveal an elevated level of alkaline phosphatase, possibly combined with elevated serum calcium (Table 15.1). Radiographic findings are variable, but radio-opacity is a feature of long-standing lesions. Histological appearance is not always helpful since differentiation from other types of fibro-osseous lesion is often difficult.

Treatment

Surgery should be deferred until after puberty when skeletal growth has ceased. It is not necessary to excise completely the

Table 15.1 Blood chemistry of bone disorders

	Calcium	Phosphate	Alkaline phosphatase
Monostotic fibrous dysplasia	N	N	N
Polyostotic fibrous dysplasia	+	N	+
Paget's disease	N	N	+ +
Hyperparathyroidism	+	−	+

N, normal; +, raised; + +, greatly raised; −, reduced

bony lesions of fibrous dysplasia and therefore a conservative surgical remodelling of the bone for cosmetic purposes is all that is required. Systemic administration of calcitonin therapy has been used in some cases.

15.2 Paget's disease (osteitis deformans)

This disorder of bone is common and has been reported as occurring in approximately 3% of individuals over the age of 40 years, although symptoms only occur in approximately 5% of these patients. The cause of the condition is unknown but involves a disturbance of bone turnover which, although predominantly resorptive in early stages, eventually results in deposition producing enlargement and increased bone density. The skull is often involved and patients may therefore complain of facial bone pain and cranial nerve defects, such as deafness or impaired vision. When the jaws are involved the maxilla is affected more frequently than the mandible. Clinical examination may reveal widening of the alveolar ridges and separation of the teeth. Difficulty may be encountered during extraction of teeth due to the presence of hypercementosis of the roots.

Diagnosis

Diagnosis is based on detection of elevated levels of serum alkaline phosphatase (Table 15.1) which isoenzyme analysis reveals to be of bony origin. Radiographs may reveal hypercementosis of the roots of the teeth.

Treatment

At the present time effective treatment involves either calcitonin, given subcutaneously, or diphosphonates, given orally.

Further reading

Eversole, L. R., Sabes, W. R. and Rovin, S. (1972) Fibrous dysplasia: a nosologic problem in the diagnosis of fibro-osseous lesions of the jaws. *Journal of Oral Pathology*, **1**, 189–220

MacDonald, D. G., Boyle, I. T. (1990) Skeletal disease. In *Oral Manifestations of Systemic Disease*, eds J. H. Jones and D. K. Mason, Baillière Tindall, London, pp. 616–659

Peacock, M. (1978) The endocrine control of calcium and phosphorus metabolism and its diseases. *Medicine*, **8**, 407–413

Smith, B. J. and Eveson, J. W. (1981) Paget's disease of bone with particular reference to dentistry. *Journal of Oral Pathology*, **10**, 223–247

Solt, D. B. (1991) The pathogenesis, oral manifestations and implications for dentistry of metabolic bone disease *Current Opinion in Dentistry*, **1**, 783–791

Chapter 16
Psychological disease

It has been estimated that approximately 10% of patients attending oral medicine outpatient clinics may have an underlying psychological disorder. Such patients complain of orofacial symptoms that do not appear to have an obvious dental cause, or request treatment that seems unreasonable. It is essential to avoid being persuaded into giving unnecessary treatment, because this often compounds the problem. It is, therefore, important that patients with psychological problems are recognized and referred for appropriate management.

It is normal to experience feelings of worry, stress, unhappiness and elation in response to different life events. These emotions are normally appropriate to the situation and resolve when the event is past. Some patients who suffer from recurrent aphthous stomatitis describe that the onset of ulcers coincides with times of stress. The mechanism by which the ulcers develop in these circumstances is not clear, but it may involve trauma due to cheek biting, which is a habit patients often develop when under stress. Parafunctional activity, such as clenching or grinding of the teeth, can also occur as a response to stress.

The distinction between a normal response to a given situation and the development of psychiatric disease is a matter of degree. When patients have a psychiatric disorder they have a mental state which is out of proportion to their overall life situation and which significantly interferes with their ability to function. Various classifications of psychiatric disorders are available, the most frequently used being either the Diagnostic and Statistical Manual (DSM) or the International Classification of Diseases (ICD-10), both of which include anxiety disorders, depressive disorders, somatoform disease and other psychological states. Simplistically, patients can be regarded as either being psychiatrically normal or having a personality disorder, a neurotic disorder or a psychotic disorder.

16.1 Anxiety

Although anxiety will be discussed as a distinct clinical entity there are those who consider psychiatric disorders, such as anxiety and depression, as being ends of a continuum of disturbance. Patients are often anxious about underlying dental treatment and it has been reported that fear of dentistry is second only to the fear of developing or having cancer. However, this type of anxiety diminishes rapidly on completion of treatment. Although such fear of dentistry is often regarded as normal in our society, it is hoped that increased emphasis on the teaching of patient management skills, usually in the context of environment, behaviour and health, will gradually improve this situation.

The main somatic manifestations of anxiety are increased muscle tension (possible factor in temporomandibular joint dysfunction) and overactivity of parasympathetic activity (bowel and urinary symptoms) and sympathetic activity (tachycardia, sweating and dry mouth). However, it is often difficult to detect anxiety clinically and therefore questionnaires have been developed to assist the clinician. The Hospital and Anxiety Depression (HAD) scale (Figure 16.1) is an assessment of anxiety which can be used for patients attending the dental surgery. The scale uses the patient's response to 14 questions, seven of which relate to anxiety and seven to depression. Questions of somatic reference, like headache or backache are deliberately avoided. Although not diagnostic in itself, the scale highlights the likelihood of anxiety or depression being present. The scale can be used repeatedly to record changes in mood over a period of time.

It is recognized that some patients experience anxiety in particular circumstances (anxiety trait), whereas others may be anxious permanently (anxiety state). It is always important to ask patients about sleep disturbance; the inability to fall asleep (early insomnia) or waking in the middle of the night (mid sleep insomnia) often accompanies anxiety. Recognition and treatment of anxiety is important in terms of orofacial diseases because it may be more appropriate to use psychological or pharmacological treatment to improve the patient's mood rather than adopting a mechanistic approach.

Anxiety neurosis

Anxiety is a normal reaction to a stressful situation and in this respect attendance at a dental surgery or out-patient clinic may involve a high degree of anxiety for some patients. Chronic anxiety may produce the complaints of xerostomia, cheek biting or bruxism.

Phobic neurosis

Phobic neurosis may be described as anxiety which occurs under certain circumstances, such as fear of lifts or spiders. Patients may have a true phobia of dental treatment and require special management.

Hysterical neurosis

Two types of hysterical neurosis, conversion and dissociative, are recognized, but there is little difference between the two and patients are likely to suffer both at the same time. In conversion neurosis an anxious patient may complain of physical symptoms, such as pain or paraesthesia with resultant relief of anxiety. Examination will often fail to reveal any abnormality. Alternatively in dissociative neurosis the patient may complain of amnesia or personality changes.

Obsessional neurosis

Obsessional personality traits are not uncommon and are characterized by recurring unnatural thoughts or impulses to perform certain behavioural acts. It is not unusual for patients to become preoccupied with the presence of coating on the teeth or the presence of halitosis. In these circumstances the patient may adopt obsessional

The Hospital Anxiety and Depression Scale

(After Zigmond and Snaith, 1983, *Acta Psychiatrica Scandinavica* 67: 361–70)

Name _____   Date: _____

This questionnaire will help you to let us know how you are. Read each item and underline the response which comes closest to how you have felt in the last few days. Don't take too long over your replies, your immediate reaction will probably be more accurate than a long thought out response.

I feel tense or 'wound up'
- Most of the time — A 3
- A lot of the time — 2
- From time to time, occasionally — 1
- Not at all — 0

I still enjoy the things I used to enjoy
- Definitely as much — D 0
- Not quite so much — 1
- Only a little — 2
- Hardly at all — 3

I get a sort of frightened feeling as if something awful is about to happen
- Very definitely and quite badly — A 3
- Yes, but not too badly — 2
- A little, but it doesn't worry me — 1
- Not at all — 0

I can laugh and see the funny side of things
- As much as I always could — D 0
- Not quite so much now — 1
- Definitely not so much now — 2
- Not at all — 3

Worrying thoughts go through my mind
- A great deal of the time — A 3
- A lot of the time — 2
- From time to time but not too often — 1
- Only occasionally — 0

I feel cheerful
- Not at all — D 3
- Not often — 2
- Sometimes — 1
- Most of the time — 0

I can sit at ease and feel relaxed
- Definitely — A 0
- Usually — 1
- Not often — 2
- Not at all — 3

I feel as if I am slowed down
- Nearly all the time — D 3
- Very often — 2
- Sometimes — 1
- Not at all — 0

I get a sort of frightened feeling like 'butterflies' in the stomach
- Not at all — A 0
- Occasionally — 1
- Quite often — 2
- Very often — 3

I have lost interest in my appearance
- Definitely — D 3
- I don't take so much care as I should — 2
- I may not take quite as much care — 1
- I take just as much care as ever — 0

I feel restless as if I have to be on the move
- Very much indeed — A 3
- Quite a lot — 2
- Not very much — 1
- Not at all — 0

I look forward with enjoyment to things
- As much as ever I did — D 0
- Rather less than I used to — 1
- Definitely less than I used to — 2
- Hardly at all — 3

I get sudden feelings of panic
- Very often indeed — A 3
- Quite often — 2
- Not very often — 1
- Not at all — 0

I can enjoy a good book or radio or TV programme
- Often — D 0
- Sometimes — 1
- Not often — 2
- Very seldom — 3

A (8–10)
D (8–10)

Fold back

This scoring device may be folded back prior to completion

Figure 16.1 HAD scale

oral hygiene procedures and the use of antiseptic mouthwashes.

Hypochondriacal neurosis

In this form of neurosis the patient is preoccupied with his or her health and is likely to present with a number of complaints. Reassurance of the absence of any clinical disease does not usually satisfy the patient, who becomes increasingly convinced that 'something has been missed'. In such circumstances it is important not to undertake unnecessary investigations or provide unnecessary treatment.

16.2 Depression

In contrast to anxiety, depression may initially present as mood disturbance. In the past, depression was viewed as either endogenous, that is with no obvious precipitating factor, or reactive in response to some major life event. This strict dichotomy has been abandoned with the realization that a combination of predisposing and precipitating factors probably occur in all patients, although the proportional contribution of each may vary. As a generalization, depression is more common in men than women and often occurs before the end of the third decade of life.

It is now well recognized that depression can manifest itself as orofacial pain, the best example being atypical facial pain. Although depressed patients may complain of a variety of sleep difficulties, early morning waking is typical. A patient who reports a sleep disturbance may also suffer loss of energy, loss of libido, loss of weight and most importantly, contemplation of suicide. Patients who are depressed typically have their period of lowest mood in the morning.

The dental practitioner should be aware of his or her patients' moods and is well placed to detect changes of mood in regular attenders. Furthermore, many dentists are familiar with the patients' home circumstances and will therefore be alert to change such as recent bereavement, which may precipitate depression.

The treatment of depression is a specialized area, and although the dental surgeon would not necessarily play a direct role in management he or she could reasonably be expected to organize the appropriate referral when indicated. Treatment options range from psychotherapy, probably in combination with drug treatment, to electroconvulsive therapy (ECT).

16.3 Schizophrenia

This common syndrome represents a fragmentation of the personality and produces altered thought, emotion perception and behaviour. Patients therefore frequently suffer delusions involving persecutory or grandiose beliefs and a hallucination of hearing voices. An example of a patient with schizophrenia is that of a 30-year-old woman who requested the removal of a post crown because she believed that metal in her mouth was acting as an aerial for the reception of messages for taxi drivers. At the time of presentation the patient had already removed many of her amalgam restorations herself with a watch-maker's drill (Plate 31). It is obvious that such a patient requires psychiatric treatment. Effective drug therapy is available and although hospitalization may be required the outcome is often good. Xerostomia can be a troublesome side-effect of the neuroleptic drug chlorpromazine, which is often used to treat schizophrenia. Provision of artificial saliva substitutes and preventive dental care can minimize these problems during the treatment period.

16.4 Anorexia nervosa and bulimia nervosa

Anorexia nervosa is characterized by vomiting and avoidance of food due to a delusion of body image where the patient sees him or herself as being obese despite the presence of emaciation. In bulimia nervosa the patient will often have normal body weight but indulge in eating binges followed by self-induced vomiting.

The repeated exposure of the teeth to regurgitated gastric acid in both these conditions leads ultimately to erosion of the tooth substance and therefore may be first detected in the dental surgery. Bilateral parotid enlargement is also a well-recognized feature of the disorder.

16.5 Dermatitis artefacta and stomatitis artefacta

A patient may deliberately produce areas of damage, either on his or her skin (dermatitis artefacta) or oral mucosa (stomatitis artefacta). The clinical appearance of such traumatic injury will depend on the manner in which they have been produced. The intra-oral lesion seen most frequently is simple cheek biting, which is seen as large areas of hyperkeratotic epithelium in the right and left buccal mucosae. In these circumstances the patient, who is usually a young anxious

individual, will sometimes admit to causing the damage and be amenable to treatment. Provision of an acrylic splint can help to break a cheek biting habit. Rarely, a patient may produce localized areas of ulceration with a finger nail, instrument or chemical substance. In this case the patient will usually deny causing the injury and diagnosis can be difficult. Similarly, if artefacting is admitted, it is often difficult to persuade such a patient to accept professional help.

Further reading

Fienmann, C. and Harris. M. (1984) Psychogenic facial pain (part I): the clinical presentation. *British Dental Journal*, **156**, 165–168

Fienmann, C. and Harris, M. (1984) Psychogenic facial pain (part II): management and prognosis *British Dental Journal*, **156**, 205–208

Harris, M. and Fienmann, C. (1990) Psychosomatic disorders. In *Oral Manifestations of Systemic Disease*, (eds J. H. Jones and D. K. Mason), Baillière Tindall, London, pp. 30–60

Hughes, A. M., Hunter, S., Still, D. and Lamey, P-J. (1989) Psychiatric disorders in a dental clinic. *British Dental Journal*, **166**, 16–19

Snaith, P. (1991) *Clinical Neurosis*, 2nd ed, Oxford Medical Publications, Oxford

Willis, J. (1979) *Lecture Notes on Psychiatry*, 5th ed, Blackwell Scientific, Oxford

Part Five
Orofacial Pain

Chapter 17
Orofacial pain

Orofacial pain is often the reason that a patient attends a dental surgery. In most cases clinical examination will reveal an obvious dental cause of pain, such as a carious tooth, lost restoration or periapical abscess, and diagnosis is straightforward. However, patients may also present with pain for which there is no apparent dental cause. Under these circumstances diagnosis has to be based on a detailed assessment of the characteristics of the symptoms (Table 17.1).

17.1 Burning mouth syndrome

The term 'burning mouth syndrome' (BMS) is used to describe the complaint of a burning sensation affecting the tongue, palate or lips. In past, terms such as glossopyrosis, glossodynia, stomatopyrosis, stomatodynia and oral dyaesthesia have been used to describe this condition. BMS predominantly affects women, but can occur in men, the female to male ratio being approximately 7:1. Generally, the older age groups are

Table 17.1 Characteristic timing and nature of the more common causes of orofacial pain

Timing of pain	Nature of pain	Condition	Comment
Present on waking	Variable	TMJ dysfunction	Associated with nocturnal bruxism or clenching
	Severe and throbbing	Migraine	Clenching may be trigger
	Severe and burning	Burning mouth syndrome (Type 2)	Needs full BMS investigations
Worse in evening	Variable	TMJ dysfunction	Associated with daytime bruxism or clenching
	Severe and burning	Burning mouth syndrome (Type 1)	Needs full BMS investigations
Coincides with eating	Diffuse pain or 'tightness'	Salivary gland obstruction	Requires sialography
	Variable	TMJ disease	Structural changes
	Sharp or boring	Giant cell arteritis	Raised ESR
	Severe, shooting, lancinating or piercing	Trigeminal neuralgia	Trigger factors
	Variable and throbbing	Pretrigeminal neuralgia	May mimic pulpitis
	Severe, shooting, lancinating or piercing	Glossopharyngeal neuralgia	Precipitated by swallowing
Disturbs sleep	Severe and episodic	Periodic migrainous neuralgia	Precipitated by alcohol
	Severe and episodic	Paroxysmal facial hemicrania	No facial flushing or running of eyes/nose
Constant	Constant, throbbing or nagging	Atypical facial pain	Exclude organic disease
	Constant and dull	Neoplasms	Requires full investigation
	Burning, gripping, boring or band-like	Psychological disorder	Requires expert assessment
	Severe and throbbing	Acute sinusitis	Increased severity on bending head forwards
Variable	Severe and burning	Burning mouth syndrome (Type 3)	Needs full BMS investigations
	Burning, gripping, boring and band-like	Psychological disorders	Requires expert assessment
	Variable	Paget's disease	Needs blood and radiographic assessment
	Intense burning	Post-herpetic neuralgia	Hyperaesthesia or paraesthesia
	Variable burning or dull	Ramsay-Hunt syndrome	Vesicles in outer ear

Adapted from Lamey, P-J. and Lewis, M.A.O. (1989) *British Dental Journal*, **167**, 385

affected, with a peak incidence in the fifth decade. Examination of the oral mucosa in BMS will fail to reveal any abnormality. Sometimes the patient may point out areas which they are concerned about, but these usually represent prominent lingual papillae or sebaceous glands.

Patients with BMS tend to describe one of three patterns of burning; type 1 – burning is not present on waking but develops as the

Table 17.2 Proposed aetiological factors in burning mouth syndrome

Vitamin B_1 deficiency
Vitamin B_2 deficiency
Vitamin B_6 deficiency
Vitamin B_{12} deficiency
Iron deficiency
Folic acid deficiency
Diabetes mellitus
Candidosis
Denture design
Xerostomia
Parafunctional habits
Cancerphobia
Anxiety
Depression
Allergy

day progresses; type 2 – burning is present on waking and persists until the patient goes to sleep; and type 3 – burning is only present intermittently and affects unusual sites, such as the throat and floor of mouth. It is useful to enquire about the pattern of symptoms, since this can be of assistance in management.

Burning mouth syndrome is a multifactorial condition with a number of recognized precipitating factors (Table 17.2). Initial management involves investigation of all potential causes and therefore a range of special tests needs to be undertaken.

Haematological investigations should exclude nutritional deficiencies and the presence of diabetes mellitus. Candidosis can be detected by the taking of smears, swabs and an oral rinse. Any dentures worn by the patients should be examined for adequate design and evidence of wear facets. Stimulated parotid flow rates should be performed if there is a clinical indication of xerostomia. Clinical examination may also support the presence of parafunctional habits, which may be seen as scalloped lateral margins of the tongue. The degree of cancerphobia can be assessed by asking the patient to rate his or her fear of the possibility of oral cancer on a scale of 0 to 10, where 0 indicates 'no

concern of cancer' and 10 indicates 'an overwhelming concern of cancer'. The presence of adverse home circumstances or life events can also be detected using a similar scale, where 0 corresponds to 'things could not be worse' and 10 indicates 'things could not be better'. This type of questioning often reveals factors such as marital problems, poor housing conditions or illness in relatives. The Hospital Anxiety and Depression (HAD) Scale can be used to determine the likelihood of the patient being anxious or depressed (see Chapter 16). If allergy is suspected in the history then referral to an appropriate specialist who will undertake patch testing is required.

Treatment

The investigation outlined above should be undertaken at the time of first presentation. Treatment should initially involve reassurance of the common nature of the problem and the absence of any serious underlying problem, in particular oral cancer. The patient should be prescribed vitamin B_1 300 mg once daily and vitamin B_6 50 mg 8-hourly for 1 month. If denture design problems exist, then the provision of new dentures should be organized. The patient should be reviewed after 4 weeks, at which time the results of haematological and microbiological tests will be available. Any abnormalities detected should be corrected with appropriate management.

Tricyclic antidepressant drug therapy has a role in the management of patients with BMS provided all other precipitating factors have been excluded. Since some tricyclic drugs have anxiolytic, antidepressant and muscle relaxant activity, they may be expected to be of benefit in patients with underlying anxiety, depression, cancerphobia or parafunctional activity. Generally the prognosis with type 1 BMS is better than type 2, because in the latter group, chronic anxiety is a particularly recalcitrant obstacle to cure. The outcome in type 3 BMS is generally good, provided that dietary or other allergic factors have been excluded. Overall, a cure rate of approximately 70% of cases with BMS should be expected. Successful management of BMS depends on assessment of all the known aetiological factors. The multifactorial nature of the condition obviously requires a team involving the dental and medical practitioner. In some patients it may be necessary to seek specialist care from an oral physician, dermatologist, psychiatrist or clinical psychologist.

17.2 Atypical facial pain

Atypical facial pain is a condition which affects women more than men and usually occurs in adults over the age of 30 years. There has been a good deal of confusion surrounding atypical facial pain, probably due to misuse of the term, which has sometimes been mistakenly interpreted as describing a pain which does not correspond to any known pain syndrome or a pain which crosses anatomical boundaries. Atypical facial pain is a distinct clinical entity with 'typical' symptoms consisting of a constant dull ache which nothing makes better or worse. The pain is chronic, being present every day from the time of waking until the patient goes to sleep. The symptoms do not waken the patient from sleep, but because the condition is strongly associated with depression, a sleep disturbance, such as early morning waking, is often present.

Although poorly localized the pain most frequently affects one side of the maxilla. Clinical examination will fail to reveal any abnormality, but radiographs of the affected region must be taken to exclude dental disease or maxillary pathology in the antrum.

Treatment

Atypical facial pain responds well to antidepressive drug therapy, dothiepin 75 mg nocte is the drug regime of choice. Alternative antidepressants may also be effective but whichever drug is chosen, therapy needs to be provided for 3–6 months. Xerostomia may be a complication of the use of antidepressant therapy.

17.3 Atypical odontalgia

This condition is closely related to atypical facial pain. The complaint is of a constant pain which is invariably localized to one tooth that is clinically and radiologically normal. The underlying cause of pain is probably similar to that of atypical facial pain.

Treatment

Treatment is based on the use of antidepressant therapy.

17.4 Periodic migrainous neuralgia (cluster headache)

Periodic migrainous neuralgia was originally considered a variant of migraine, but is probably a separate clinical entity. The condition affects males more than females and does not usually occur under the age of 20 years. The term 'periodic' is included in the description of the disorder because attacks are episodic. Periodic migrainous neuralgia is one of the few orofacial pain conditions which can wake a patient from sleep, a factor which is helpful in diagnosis.

Symptoms can develop within minutes and are described by patients as being severe. Pain is often centred around the orbital region and it is thought the condition may arise from within the internal carotid circulation. Autonomic symptoms, such as conjunctival injection, rhinorrhoea and lacrimation, often accompany the pain, but it is still unclear what mechanisms underlie these features. The headache generally lasts for 30–90 minutes and can disappear almost as quickly as it arose. Although specific trigger factors can rarely be identified, some patients report that alcohol, even in very small amounts, can precipitate an attack.

Several studies have been undertaken to try to explain the mechanism of pain and autonomic dysfunction in periodic migrainous neuralgia. Thermographic investigation has shown that there is an asymmetrical temperature pattern over the supraorbital vessels in some patients, which suggests that the boundary region between internal and external carotid arteries could be of importance. An abnormality of the internal carotid artery at the level of the carotid canal could produce hypersensitivity of terminal vessels due to oedema, which may in turn damage surrounding sympathetic nerve fibres by compression. A possible role of hormones, enkephalins and endorphins has been suggested due to the periodicity of the disorder and predominance in males, but as yet this is not proved. The trigeminal nerve may also have a role because destruction of the gasserian ganglion produces relief in the great majority of sufferers.

Treatment

At the present time periodic migrainous neuralgia is largely treated with anti-inflammatory drugs. Indomethacin taken prophylactically at a dose of 75 mg, can control and prevent the occurrence of symptoms. The duration of prophylactic treatment is uncertain but a course of 3 months is effective in the most chronic cases. Clearly, if a precipitatory factor, such as alcohol, has been identified then this needs to be avoided.

17.5 Paroxysmal facial hemicrania

Paroxysmal facial hemicrania is characterized by a pain very similar to that of periodic migrainous neuralgia, but can be regarded as a separate condition because autonomic dysfunction is absent. Furthermore, the symptoms may be chronic, occurring every day rather than paroxysmal. A dull throbbing pain is the predominant complaint, but attacks are not all of equal severity and a severe jabbing pain may develop. Paroxysmal facial hemicrania always affects one side (hemicrania) and tends to be of short duration, lasting between 15 and 20 minutes. Patients can have several attacks in one day and are rarely woken during sleep.

Treatment

Prophylactic indomethacin (75 mg nocte) is the treatment of choice.

17.6 Tension headache

Tension headache is an ill-defined condition, but in clinical practice is to some extent a diagnosis of exclusion. The term can be applied if the complaint consists of a tightness, pressure or constriction of variable intensity, frequency and duration. Tension is the most common cause of headache and affects males and females equally. Precise epidemiological information is not available because many patients are not likely to seek treatment, but it has been estimated that in some countries 5–10% of the population suffer from a tension headache at least once a week.

The headache may not always be suboccipital and indeed about 30% of patients say the whole head is involved. Unlike most pain syndromes the condition is not of sufficient severity to interfere with work or other activities.

Treatment

Commonly prescribed or over-the-counter medicines usually alleviate the headache.

17.7 Migraine

Migraine is a clinical diagnosis based on the presence of a severe prolonged headache (hours or days), associated with nausea and vomiting. The patient may suffer heightened sensitivity to external stimuli, such as light (photophobia), noise (phonophobia) or smell (osmophobia). Dietary factors, such as alcohol, chocolate, cheese or citrus fruits, can trigger attacks. In almost three-quarters of cases of migraine there is a family history of the disorder. The condition is slightly more common in women than men and can occur at any age but usually develops in the second and third decades of life.

Treatment

The response of migraine to agents such as aspirin, paracetamol, pizotifen, propanolol or ergotamine is variable, and therefore individual patients usually try a variety of treatments before discovering which is best for them. From an aetiological point of view, the fact that the headache tends to start in the morning or soon after, has led to the use of acrylic splint therapy. The acrylic splint should completely cover the occlusal surfaces of the upper or lower teeth (Plate 32) and only be worn at night. Approximately 80% of patients who suffer migraine on waking can be relieved of their symptoms entirely following this approach. A major advantage of splint therapy is that it avoids the need for systemic anti-migraine drug therapy.

17.8 Temporomandibular joint dysfunction syndrome (TMJ dysfunction)

There has probably been more written about TMJ dysfunction than any other facial pain syndrome, but it remains one of the major areas of divided opinion concerning cause and treatment. The confusion may in part be due to the variety of terms that have been used to describe the complaint, which has included facial pain dysfunction, myofacial pain dysfunction and facial arthromyalgia. Regardless of terminology most authors are agreed on the main symptoms, which consist of a constant dull unilateral or bilateral pre-auricular/auricular pain which can undergo

acute exacerbations radiating into the temple, maxilla or occipital regions. In addition, the patient is likely to complain of trismus, limited jaw movements, audible 'click' on opening, tenderness of the joint and headache. When dealing with TMJ pain it is important to differentiate between TMJ dysfunction which involves abnormal physical activity of the joint and TMJ diseases in which there is a pathological change of the joint (see below). The cause of TMJ dysfunction remains uncertain, but is likely to involve occlusal abnormalities, lack of posterior teeth, parafunctional clenching habits, nocturnal bruxism, anxiety and depression. In some cases the patient may be aware of an acute incident of local trauma whilst eating or yawning which initiated the problem.

Examination of the patient is likely to reveal tenderness of one or both of the temporomandibular joints and associated muscles of mastication. There may well be an audible click on jaw movement. The patient's dentition may show evidence of bruxism, wear facets or lack of posterior teeth. Radiographic examination of the joints is usually unnecessary because in the majority of cases there is no visible abnormality. Diagnosis is made from the clinical history and examination.

Treatment

Opinions on the treatment of TMJ dysfunction are widely divided, but there is little doubt that splint therapy has a major role. A number of splint designs have been suggested, but experience would support the use of full occlusal coverage. An acrylic splint with approximately 2 mm opening and clasps is the most effective approach. The decision to construct either an upper or lower splint is based on the number and position of the patient's remaining teeth. In acute or severe cases the patient should be provided with a mild anxiolytic and muscle relaxant, such as diazepam. Alternatively, the use of tricyclic antidepressant therapy, in particular dothiepin, has been found to produce symptomatic improvement.

17.9 Temporomandibular joint disease (TMJ disease)

The vast majority of patients who complain of pain associated with the temporomandibular joint have TMJ dysfunction. There are, however, a number of pathological conditions which may produce anatomical changes in the joint. It is generally accepted that the temporomandibular joint is often involved in patients with rheumatoid arthritis. Radiographic examination of the joints using tomography or a transpharyngeal view in patients with rheumatoid arthritis may reveal erosions, proliferations or flattening of the condylar heads. It may also be helpful to undertake arthrography (injection of contrast medium into the joint space) or arthroscopy (direct visualization of the joint surface using endoscopy). More recently, computed tomography and magnetic resonance imaging have been used to detect joint abnormalities.

Treatment

A conservative approach using splint therapy with or without drug therapy will produce symptomatic improvement in many patients. In some patients however it will be necessary to consider a surgical approach to correct gross structural abnormalities.

17.10 Trigeminal neuralgia

The pain of trigeminal neuralgia is characteristic, in that it is limited to the anatomical pathways or one of three branches of the trigeminal nerve. The condition is slightly more common in women than men and rarely occurs before the age of 40 years. The pain is severe, and is described as being shooting, lancinating or piercing in nature. Sufferers may describe trigger spots on their skin or in their mouth, whilst others report that smiling, eating or washing can bring on an attack.

Clinical examination of patients will not reveal any abnormality except if a trigger spot or precipitating movement is present. Histological study from autopsy material has suggested that trigeminal neuralgia may arise as a result of areas of demyelination along the distribution of the trigeminal nerve.

Other studies have suggested that patients have an aberrant intracranial artery in the cerebello-pontine region. It is rare to find accompanying organic disease, but it should be appreciated that neoplasms of the nasopharynx, maxillary antrum and middle ear, and aneurysms have occasionally been described in association with the disease and therefore should be excluded. Trigeminal neuralgia occurring in patients under the age of 40 years suggests the presence of an underlying systemic disease, in particular multiple sclerosis or HIV infection.

Treatment

Trigeminal neuralgia can be successfully treated medically with carbamazepine. Initially, a dose of 100–200 mg daily should be given and increased every 3–4 days by 100 mg until pain control is achieved. In practice, a dose of 400–600 mg is usually sufficient to control the pain. The half-life of carbamazepine varies depending on the frequency of dosage prescribed, and therefore the more frequently the drug is administered the shorter the half-life. If a regimen of divided doses fails to control the pain it is worthwhile trying a single dose approach. The duration of treatment remains speculative but most patients can gradually reduce therapy after 6–12 symptom-free months. Prescribing the drug for short periods of time (1–2 months) will almost certainly result in a recurrence of pain. Although side-effects of carbamazepine therapy are uncommon, it is advisable to undertake a baseline full blood count and measure levels of liver enzymes. These tests should be repeated at approximately 3-monthly intervals whilst treatment is being given.

If carbamazepine therapy is found to be ineffective or has to be discontinued because of side-effects then consideration can be given to the use of phenytoin, clonazepam or oxcarbamazepine, (a newer analogue of carbamazepine not presently available on general prescription). Should all types of medical therapy fail then surgical treatment may have to be considered. Cryotherapy, surgical section, fractional rhizotomy and thermocoagulation have all been tried with varying success. Unfortunately, surgical techniques produce permanent facial anaesthesia or dysaesthia which can be troublesome to the patient. In addition, section of one root of the trigeminal nerve may lead to recurrence of the condition in one of the other divisions of the nerve.

17.11 Pretrigeminal neuralgia

There is some debate concerning the existence of this condition, but it is generally accepted that trigeminal neuralgia may be preceded by symptoms which are described as being like toothache. It has been proposed that up to 20% of patients who develop trigeminal neuralgia have previously suffered from these symptoms, which have therefore been described as pretrigeminal neuralgia.

Clinical and radiographical examination will fail to reveal any abnormality and the pain of pretrigeminal neuralgia may therefore be confused with pulpitis, periapical pathology or cracked tooth syndrome.

Treatment

Pretrigeminal neuralgia responds to carbamazepine therapy, and this agent should be given in cases where there is doubt that a pain is of dental origin.

17.12 Glossopharyngeal neuralgia

The pain of glossopharyngeal neuralgia is identical to trigeminal neuralgia, but is usually initiated by swallowing and the pain itself is located in the throat or tonsillar area, larynx or ear. As with trigeminal neuralgia the presence of organic disease, such as a pharyngeal carcinoma, should be excluded.

Treatment

Carbamazepine is usually successful in controlling the pain. Surgical options are available if the condition is unresponsive to drug therapy.

17.13 Giant cell arteritis

Giant cell arteritis is a condition which was previously termed temporal arteritis. The latter is not a good term because the condition can affect vessels in the head or neck other than the temporal artery. The condition generally occurs in individuals over the age of 60 years and is more common in women than men. It is one of the few facial pain syndromes in which patients describe systemic upset, including weight loss, muscle weakness and lethargy, although muscle biopsy, enzymology and electromyography are normal. The basic pathological changes of giant cell arteritis appear to be of a granulomatous arteritis. The pain can be brought on by eating and therefore the patient can only eat for short periods before resting to allow the pain to subside. This limitation of normal eating is thought to be ischaemic in origin and has been misnamed 'jaw claudication'. Blood investigations will often show a raised erythrocyte sedimentation rate (ESR). It has been proposed that temporal artery biopsy is of value in confirming the diagnosis but the granulomatous lesions occur sporadically along the vessel (skip lesions) and therefore several biopsies may be required to detect them. More importantly, the delay in obtaining the results of such a biopsy can be hazardous as blindness is a recognized complication of untreated giant cell arteritis.

Treatment

The treatment of choice in giant cell arteritis is oral prednisolone at a dose of 40–60 mg daily in divided doses. After symptoms have been controlled the therapy can be reduced, although a low maintenance dose may be required for 3–6 months. The ESR is a reasonable guide to disease activity and this should fall to normal levels (less than 20 mm/h) following institution of steroid therapy.

Further reading

Fienmann, C., Harris, M. and Cawley, R. (1984) Psychogenic facial pain: presentation and treatment. *British Medical Journal*, **288**, 436–439

Lamey, P-J., Lamb, A. B. (1988) Prospective study of the aetiological factors in burning mouth syndrome. *British Medical Journal*, **296**, 1243–1246

Lamey, P-J. and Lewis, M. A. O. (1989) Oral medicine in practice: orofacial pain. *British Dental Journal*, **167**, 384–389

Seymour, R. A. (1983) Dental Pain 3: The measurement of pain. *Dental Update*, **10**, 446–454

Watts, P., Peret, K. and Juniper, R. (1986) Migraine and temporomandibular joint: the final answer? *British Dental Journal*, **161**, 170–175

Zakrzewska, J. M. (1990) Medical management of trigeminal neuralgia. *British Dental Journal*, **168**, 399–401

Zakrzewska, J. M. (1991) Surgical management of trigeminal neuralgia. *British Dental Journal*, **170**, 61–62

Part Six
Salivary Gland Disease

Chapter 18
Salivary gland disease

The salivary tissue consists of three paired major glands (parotid, submandibular and sublingual) within the neck and numerous minor glands which are distributed throughout the oral mucosa. Disorders can be localized to an individual gland or widespread throughout all the glands. Salivary gland disease can result in reduced production of saliva, which in turn may produce a number of oral symptoms.

18.1 Developmental abnormalities

Formation of the salivary glands begins at an early stage of embryonic life (4–12 weeks) as invaginations of the oral epithelium which subsequently differentiate into the ducts and acinar tissue. Despite the complex anatomy of the orofacial region, developmental disturbances involving the salivary glands are rare. When a salivary abnormality does occur it is usually accompanied by other defects, such as anophthalmia, cleft palate or absence of the lacrimal glands.

Aplasia/agenesis

The congenital absence of one or more of the major salivary glands is termed either aplasia or agenesis. It is extremely uncommon but if present appears to involve the parotid glands predominately. Other abnormalities, such as occlusion or absence of the salivary ducts, are also rare, but have been described within the sublingual and submandibular glands. Hypoplasia of salivary tissue probably occurs, but is unlikely to produce any noticeable clinical symptoms.

Diagnosis

Sialography is a useful way of demonstrating the presence of suspected major structural defects either of salivary ducts or the glands themselves. Surprisingly, xerostomia does not appear to be a major clinical problem in these patients, but any reduction in salivary flow from birth will predispose to a number of oral complaints in later life.

Treatment

Management of xerostomia is based on providing artificial saliva substitutes, minimizing dental disease by preventive measures and treating opportunistic infections, such as oral candidosis and bacterial sialadenitis.

Aberrancy

Additional or aberrant salivary glands are rare but may be found at a variety of abnormal sites, including the mandible, base of neck, mastoid bone and lymphoid tissue. Aberrant tissue occurring at the angle of the mandible has been associated with a radiolucent area which may be seen at this site (Stafne bone cyst).

Diagnosis

Sialography may be helpful in confirming the presence of salivary tissue in this situation.

Treatment

Aberrant salivary tissue in areas distant from the head and neck does not usually represent a clinical problem, but should not be overlooked as a potential site of tumour formation.

18.2 Other abnormalities

Salivary calculus (sialolith)

Development of one or more calcified deposits, known as calculi or sialoliths, within salivary gland ducts is not uncommon. The composition of these structures is approximately two-thirds inorganic, mainly calcium and phosphate, with neutral lipids accounting for the organic content. Although the majority of calculi occur in major salivary glands, particularly the submandibular, they may occur within the ducts of minor glands. The cause of calculus formation is not fully understood, but it has been proposed that fungi, bacteria or desquamating epithelium cells can act as an initial nucleus of progressive calcification.

Salivary calculi are usually asymptomatic until they cause obstruction of the duct which will produce pain and swelling of the affected gland. Patients often report transitory periods (1–2 hours) of gland swelling and discomfort, especially at mealtimes. If untreated at this stage, progressive blockage of the duct is likely to predispose to an acute bacterial sialadenitis with symptoms of persistent pain, swelling and possibly pyrexia.

Diagnosis

Clinically, there may be no abnormality at the time of examination, although stimulation of salivary flow may produce obvious extra-oral swelling of the affected gland. Intraorally a calcified deposit may be seen at the duct orifice (Plate 33) or may be palpable within the duct. Radiography is helpful in confirming the diagnosis and may reveal the presence of multiple lesions (Figure 18.1). However, not all calculi are radiopaque and therefore sialography, which will also detect the presence of mucous plugs, may be required.

Treatment

At the present time, surgical removal of salivary calculi is the treatment of choice. If the deposits are present at the anterior part of the duct or its orifice, then a temporary suture should be placed distal to the calculus to prevent any posterior displacement during removal. A scalpel or dissecting scissors may be used to open the roof of the duct to

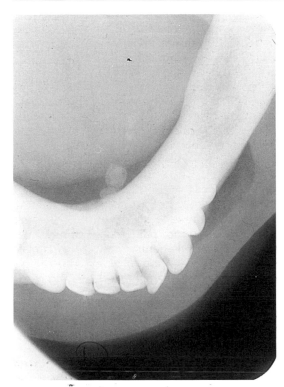

Figure 18.1 Occlusal radiograph of sialoliths in the submandibular duct

gain access to the calculus. It is often preferable to either leave the wound open or suture the edges to adjacent mucosa because attempts at complete closure are likely to result in occlusion of the duct lumen. Consideration has to be given to removal of the gland when the calculus is either positioned distally in the duct or within the gland itself. Intraglandular calculi, particularly those occurring in the submandibular gland, can reach a surprisingly large size without producing clinical symptoms and therefore are occasionally first detected as an incidental finding on radiographs.

Sialography should be performed 2–3 weeks after the removal of any calculus to determine the presence of structural gland damage. There is evidence from salivary studies using scintiscanning that a previous history of calculi within the submandibular duct does not result in a permanent reduction of gland function. The same is probably not true of the parotid gland, which unlike the submandibular gland, is composed mainly of serious acinar cells which are likely to undergo atrophy under back-pressure.

A lithotripter has been successfully used experimentally for the disintegration of salivary calculi and this form of treatment may be an alternative to surgery in the future.

Papillary or duct stricture

Inflammatory oedema or fibrosis due to acute or chronic trauma to the duct papilla will compromise the duct lumen and therefore limit salivary flow. Anatomical strictures may occur at any other site along major ducts, although the cause of the majority of these defects is unknown at the present time.

The buccinator window anomaly is an example of a physiological stricture specific to the region where the parotid duct penetrates the buccinator muscle. The condition is rare and it is believed that spasm of the buccinator muscle effectively occludes the lumen of the duct, which in turn will produce swelling of the gland itself.

Patients suffering from either anatomical or physiological strictures characteristically complain of the rapid development of a salivary gland swelling during eating which subsequently resolves over a period of 1–2 hours. However, the absence of gland swelling does not exclude salivary gland obstruction being present.

Diagnosis

Sialography is required to determine the site and extent of any stricture. Pressure-monitored sialography is the only way of diagnosing a physiological stricture of the duct, because although the sialogram will appear normal, filling pressure will be raised during initial introduction of contrast medium.

Treatment

Performance of sialography on a gland with a stricture is often sufficient to produce dilatation and symptomatic improvement. If symptoms persist and the defect is in the anterior part of the duct then further dilatation may be performed using lacrimal probes. No satisfactory treatment for the buccinator window anomaly has yet been developed.

The presence of neoplasia in adjacent structures should be excluded whenever a stricture of a salivary gland duct is thought to be the result of external duct compression.

Mucocele

Mucocele is a term describing a common salivary 'cyst' involving minor salivary glands tissue. Two types have been described, mucous retention and mucous extravasation, although differentiation is not possible clinically. Diagnosis is made by histological examination of an excised lesion which will reveal either a pool of mucous saliva in the tissue surrounded by connective tissue (extravasation) type or, more rarely, a cyst cavity lined by epithelium (retention type). The term 'ranula' is applied to a retention type of mucocele which affects the sublingual gland. The cause of a mucocele is uncertain, but it has been suggested that trauma to excretory ducts is likely to be involved.

Diagnosis

A mucocele characteristically presents as a painless fluctuant submucosal swelling, often with a blue coloration (Plate 34). Although the lesion may develop at any intraoral site, the lip, especially the lower lip, is most often involved. The lesion is usually persistent, but some patients refer to their complaint as a 'recurring blister', which periodically swells and discharges.

Treatment

Treatment consists of either complete excision by careful blunt dissection or the application of a cryoprobe (three applications of 1-minute duration with recovery period of 1-minute between each application). Whichever method of treatment is employed, the patient should be warned of the likelihood of recurrence, particularly when surgical excision is thought to be incomplete. Patients should also be aware that damage to nerves during surgical removal of a mucocele occurring in the lower lip may produce a transient paraesthesia of the mental nerve.

A ranula is usually larger than a mucocele and therefore treatment is based on surgical marsupialization. An attempt to achieve enucleation is likely to be unsuccessful due to the poorly defined margins of the lesion.

18.3 Infections

Bacterial sialadenitis

Acute suppurative sialadenitis was previously a frequent complication in hospitalized patients, especially following abdominal surgery. The use of prophylactic antibiotics and a better understanding of fluid balance has resulted in a marked reduction in the incidence of this infection as a postoperative complaint. However, bacterial sialadenitis may still occur in association with either a localized or systemic cause of reduced salivary flow. The cause is not fully understood, but it is generally assumed to involve an ascending bacterial infection of members of the oral microflora, usually a mixture of facultative streptococci and strictly anaerobic bacteria.

Diagnosis

Acute suppurative sialadenitis presents as an acutely painful swelling of the affected gland accompanied by a discharge of pus at the main duct orifice. An aspirated sample of pus should be obtained by placing a fine polythene catheter in the duct; a microbiological swab of the discharge is likely to be contaminated by mixed saliva. Antibiotic sensitivity should be routinely requested along with identity of microorganisms. However, because the results of culture and sensitivity tests may not be available for 2–3 days, the initial choice of therapy may have to be based on information obtained from a Gram stain of the pus sample.

Rare bacterial causes of suppurative sialadenitis include actinomycosis, gonorrhoea, syphilis and tuberculosis.

Treatment

Antibiotic therapy should be commenced, with amoxycillin as the agent of first choice. A loading dose of 3 g amoxycillin may be prescribed prior to conventional therapy of 250 mg 8-hourly for 4–5 days. Alternatively, erythromycin may be prescribed for patients with a hypersensitivity to the penicillin group. If the infection is clearly secondary to the presence of calculus then this should be removed surgically at an early stage to allow drainage of pus. Following resolution of acute symptoms, sialography should be performed on the affected gland to detect the presence of any predisposing factors, such as calculi, mucous plugs or benign structures.

Chronic recurrent parotitis of childhood

Chronic recurrent parotitis of childhood is characterized by repeated episodes of suppurative sialadenitis affecting the parotid glands. No obvious predisposing factors are present.

Diagnosis

Sialography of the affected glands will demonstrate bilateral sialectasis although clinical symptoms usually affect one gland only. There is some evidence that sialectasis may resolve in later life.

Treatment

The condition may require long-term antibiotic therapy, but symptoms generally resolve around the time of puberty.

Viral sialadenitis

The mumps virus, a paramyxovirus, is the most common viral infection involving the salivary glands. Characteristically, the parotid glands are affected, although in about 10% of cases the submandibular glands may be involved either alone or in addition to the parotid glands. The incubation period of infection is 2–3 weeks, during which time the virus can be detected in the saliva. The highly infective nature of the saliva at this stage probably accounts for outbreaks which occur within communities. In addition to salivary gland swelling, patients may complain of fever, malaise and headache. In adulthood, orchitis or oophoritis represents a serious complication which may lead to sterility.

Diagnosis

Diagnosis of mumps is usually made relatively easily by the characteristic clinical symptoms and signs. However, it should be confirmed by the demonstration of antibodies to nucleoprotein core (soluble or S-antigen) or protein coat (viral or V-antigen) of the virus particle. Evidence of recent infection is supported by significant levels of IgM antibody to both S and V antigens. Although levels of antibody to the V antigen may persist for many years the amounts of S antigen fall rapidly after clinical resolution.

Treatment

No specific treatment is available, but symptoms usually subside within 1 week.

18.4 Decreased salivation

Sjögren's syndrome

Since Sjögren first described an association between dry mouth, dry eyes and rheumatoid arthritis, a variety of diagnostic criteria for Sjögren's syndrome have evolved. It is generally accepted that two forms, primary and secondary, exist. Primary Sjögren's syndrome, previously referred to as Sicca syndrome, consists of dry eyes and dry mouth. In the secondary form, the patient has a connective tissue disorder in addition to suffering from dry eyes and/or dry mouth. Sjögren's syndrome is a relatively common condition and it has been estimated that approximately 15% of patients with rheumatoid arthritis are affected.

Although rheumatoid arthritis is the most frequent connective tissue disease component, other conditions including systemic lupus erythematosis, progressive systemic sclerosis or primary biliary cirrhosis may be involved.

Malignant lymphoma is a well-recognized complication in patients with Sjögren's syndrome, particularly the primary variant and those who have persistent parotid swelling.

Diagnosis

Diagnosis of Sjögren's syndrome is based on results of a number of tests, including stimulated parotid salivary flow rates, lacrimal flow rates (Schirmer test), labial gland biopsy, sialography and immunological studies (Table 18.1). Labial gland biopsy, the single most specific diagnostic criterion, should involve five or more lobules, because not all lobules show features of the condition. In addition, the minor glands should be taken from an area of the lip with apparently normal overlying mucosa, because inflammatory changes may be seen in minor glands underlying mucosal abnormalities. Sialography will usually demonstrate sialectasis, although 'false positives' can occur when a hand injection technique rather than a physiological method of introducing the contrast medium is used.

Treatment

Treatment of the oral component of Sjögren's syndrome essentially consists of alleviating the symptoms of xerostomia, treating candidal infection and preventing dental caries and periodontal disease.

Table 18.1 Features of primary or secondary Sjögren's syndrome (SS)

Stimulated parotid salivary flow rate	Less than 0.7 ml/min
Lacrimal flow rate (Schirmer test)	Less than 5 mm wetting/5 min
Labial gland biopsy	Focal lymphocytic infiltrate Duct dilatation Acinar loss Periductal fibrosis
Sialography	Sialectasis
Serology	Rheumatoid factor (positive in 90% of patients) Antinuclear factor (positive in 50% of patients) Anti-salivary duct (positive in 50% of patients) Anti-Ro (SS-A/SjD) and Anti-La (SS-B/SjT) (positive in 50–80% of primary SS patients)

Parotid biopsies from patients with Sjögren's syndrome, which have previously been reported as benign lymphoepithelial lesion and now referred to by some as myoepithelial sialadenitis, may progress to B-cell lymphomas. The transition to a lymphomatous state can be accompanied by a reduction in circulating auto-antibody titres, and therefore serial titres may be helpful.

Xerostomia

Many patients complain of a dry mouth although their salivary gland function is often found to be normal. True xerostomia may either be due to a primary salivary gland disease or a secondary manifestation of a systemic disorder or drug therapy. Primary salivary gland diseases include Sjögren's syndrome, postirradiation damage or developmental anomalies. Secondary systemic causes of xerostomia include chronic anxiety states, dehydration or drug therapy (Table 18.2).

Diagnosis

Confirmation of reduced salivary production is based on clinical examination and measurement of salivary flow rates.

Treatment

Patients with xerostomia will complain of a number of oral symptoms, especially

Table 18.2 Types of drugs which may produce xerostomia

Antidepressants
Antihistamines
Anticholinergic drugs
Potent diuretics
Hypotensive agents
Muscle relaxants
Narcotics
Hypnotics
Neuroleptics (major tranquillizers)
Sympathomimetics

difficulty in talking or swallowing, poor retention of dentures and generalized oral discomfort. A range of salivary substitutes, based on either methyl cellulose or mucin, are available to alleviate the reduction in saliva. Sialogues, such as glycerine and lemon preparations, should be restricted to edentulous patients because frequent use will encourage dental caries in dentate individuals. Rigorous oral hygiene measures and preventive regimens such as topical fluoride therapy should be instituted because reduced amounts of saliva will predispose to an increased incidence of caries, periodontal disease and oral infection, particularly candidosis. Dietary advice should be given, especially concerning the limitation of sugar intake.

18.5 Increased salivation
Sialorrhoea

Increased salivation (sialorrhoea, ptyalism) is a relatively uncommon complaint compared with that of a dry mouth. Transient periods of excessive salivation do occur in association with painful oral ulcerative conditions, such as primary herpetic gingivostomatitis or recurrent oral ulceration. It may be a complaint in patients provided with dentures or an orthodontic appliance for the first time. Drooling is a well-recognized problem in patients with a neurological disturbance particularly mental retardation, Parkinson's disease, schizophrenia and epilepsy. Rarer causes of excess salivation include mercury poisoning, acrodynia, rabies and drug therapy (Table 18.3).

Table 18.3 Types of drugs which may produce sialorrhoea

Anticholinesterases
Ethionamide
Iodides
Ketamine
Mercurials
Niridazole

Diagnosis

In otherwise healthy patients with no obvious predisposing factors, a complaint of 'saliva pouring out of the mouth' or 'soaking the pillows at night' is likely to indicate a psychological basis. In such circumstances, appropriate psychological assessment and treatment are required.

Treatment

No specific treatment is available for sialorrhoea. However, management of any underlying psychological illness usually leads to symptomatic improvement.

18.6 Sialosis

Sialosis is defined as non-inflammatory, non-neoplastic swelling of salivary glands. The parotid glands are most frequently involved bilaterally; the submandibular or sublingual glands may sometimes be affected. The cause of the swelling is not fully understood, although it has been associated with a number of systemic diseases, particularly diabetes mellitus, acromegaly, alcoholism, malnutrition, bulimia nervosa and anorexia nervosa. Sialosis has also been described as a side-effect of a number of drugs (Table 18.4).

Diagnosis

Investigation of patients with sialosis should include determination of levels of venous plasma blood glucose, growth hormone and liver function tests. A recent history of drug therapy should be excluded. Palatal erosions on the upper anterior teeth are suggestive of anorexia nervosa or bulimia nervosa.

Treatment

If potential aetiological factors are detected then corrective treatment usually results in some reduction of salivary gland swelling. However, in some patients the cause of persistent salivary gland swelling is not found. In such cases gland biopsy may be helpful to exclude the possibility of uncommon conditions, such as sarcoidosis, leukaemic infiltrates and adenolymphoma.

18.7 Neoplasms

Neoplasms arising in the salivary glands are relatively uncommon, accounting for approximately 3% of all neoplasms. However, in the oral cavity, salivary neoplasms are second only to squamous cell carcinoma arising in the mucosa. Many types of tumours or neoplasms both benign and malignant are recognized (Table 18.5). The parotid gland is affected ten times more frequently than other glands with pleomorphic adenoma, accounting for approximately 75% of neoplasms at this site. Although less common, neoplasms arising in

Table 18.4 Drugs which may produce sialosis

Anti-thyroid agents
Insulin
Iodides
Isoprenaline
Methyldopa
Oxyphenbutazone
Phenylbutazone
Sulphonamides

Table 18.5 Important salivary gland neoplasms

Benign lesions
    Pleomorphic adenoma ('mixed tumour')
    Adenolymphoma (Warthin's tumour)
    Oxyphilic adenoma

Malignant lesions
    Mucoepidermoid carcinoma
    Acinic cell carcinoma
    Adenoid cystic carcinoma
    Adenocarcinoma
    Epidermoid carcinoma
    Undifferentiated carcinoma

the minor salivary glands are more worrying because approximately 50% of lesions at this site are malignant.

Diagnosis

Minor salivary gland neoplasms usually present as painless swellings or areas of ulceration affecting the palate or lip. Fortunately, lesions at this site are usually relatively small and can undergo excisional biopsy to confirm diagnosis. Neoplasms arising in the parotid, submandibular or sublingual gland present as progressively enlarging swellings. A presentation of facial nerve palsy in addition to parotid swelling is highly suggestive of the presence of a malignant neoplasm. In addition, persistent salivary gland pain, an infrequent clinical complaint, should be regarded as suspicious because even small neoplasms can produce degrees of discomfort. Neoplasms of the major salivary glands can be investigated in some detail preoperatively using sialography, CT-sialography or magnetic resonance imaging. Such techniques will not only determine the presence of a space-occupying lesion but will suggest its origin and extent. Therefore this type of presurgical approach is becoming routine in centres involved in the management of salivary gland disease.

The condition of necrotizing sialometaplasia can produce a diagnostic problem when considering the presence of minor salivary gland tumours, especially in the palate where it may mimic squamous cell carcinoma both clinically and histologically. Necrotizing sialometaplasia is of unknown cause although preceding trauma, including dental treatment, infection and ischaemia have been suggested as important factors. Although worrying initially, the lesion is self-limiting and will resolve within 7–10 days.

Treatment

Surgery is the treatment of choice for salivary gland neoplasms at any site because the lesions are radioresistant. Radiotherapy should be considered as a palliative form of management rather than as curative treatment. Even if a neoplasm is benign, complete excision is indicated because any residual lesion will inevitably enlarge and there is a risk of malignant change (carcinoma ex pleomorphic salivary adenoma).

As with any neoplasm, patients with salivary gland lesions require long-term follow-up to exclude the possibility of recurrence.

18.8 Salivary gland investigations

Sialometry

Sialometry is the measurement of salivary flow rates which may be assessed either as resting or stimulated. Consideration has to be given to the time of day the sample was obtained and the type of stimulant used. The relative values of stimulated and unstimulated salivary flow rates have been debated, but most information is based on stimulated parotid flow rates. Collection of saliva from the parotid glands is achieved by the use of a Carlsson-Crittenden cup placed over each duct orifice (Plate 35). Flow is stimulated by placement of 1 ml of 10% citric acid on the dorsum of the tongue. A flow of at least 0.7 ml/min would be considered normal. Measurement of flow rates of the submandibular gland is more complicated and is usually used only for research purposes.

Sialochemistry

The analysis of salivary constituents has been applied in the study of a variety of disease states and abnormalities have been detected in patients with sarcoidosis, Sjögren's syndrome and a variety of hormonal disorders. The technique is not in widespread diagnostic use but can be used to measure and monitor levels of certain drugs and hormones.

Rheology

To date, little clinical information is available on the rheological properties of saliva, but it has been suggested that alterations in flow and consistency may be involved in the perception of xerostomia and taste.

Sialography

Sialography is a method of direct demonstration of the duct network of either the submandibular or parotid salivary gland. Occasionally, the sublingual gland may be visualized, but this is a chance occurrence. The technique is based on the infusion of a radio-opaque contrast medium into the main salivary duct. Contrast media are available with either an oil or water base. Contrast media based on poppy-seed oil were originally used routinely for sialography. However, it has been recommended that oil-based media should no longer be used because of problems of overfilling of the gland which can lead to loss of duct archi-

tecture on the radiograph, retention of media within the gland and gland damage. Water-based media containing sodium and meglumine salts of diatrizoic acid and iothalamic acid do not have these problems and are now the contrast agent of choice.

Methods of introducing the medium include hand-held injection, hydrostatic pressure or continuous infusion. The hand-held technique carries a risk of producing high pressure within the gland which may cause pain and gland damage. The hydrostatic method overcomes the problems of excessive infusion pressure, but may not achieve adequate gland filling in obstructive disorders. Continuous-infusion pressure-monitored (CIPM) is the preferred method since it allows accurate control of infusion and has the advantage of alerting the clinician to the presence of excessive filling pressure. The equipment required for CIPM sialography is represented in Figure 18.2. A sterile polythene cannula is inserted into the excretory duct orifice. It may be necessary to use an infiltration of local anaesthetic in the

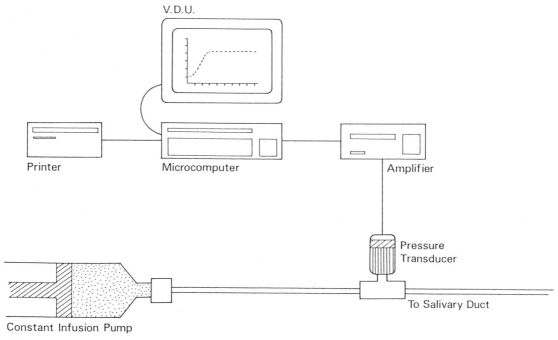

Figure 18.2 Equipment required for CIPM sialography

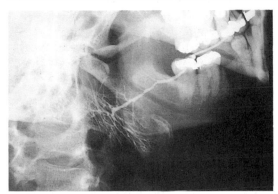

Figure 18.3 Sialogram of the right parotid gland showing strictures in the main excretory duct

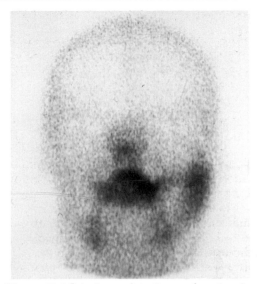

Figure 18.4 Scintiscan showing no function in the right parotid gland

floor of the mouth when the submandibular gland is being investigated. A water-based medium should be infused at a rate of 0.5 ml/min. Radiographs are taken between 2 and 4 minutes and should include two views in different planes: usually a lateral oblique and anteroposterior view. A 15° oblique lateral view is also occasionally required when the submandibular gland is being investigated.

Sialography is an invaluable method of demonstrating structural abnormalities, particularly benign strictures, mucous plugs and calculi (Figure 18.3). Distribution of the contrast medium may produce distinctive radiographic features in the presence of a chronic inflammatory condition within the salivary glands. This is particularly true for the duct dilation (sialodochiectasis) and peripheral collections of medium (sialectasis) seen during the sialography of the parotid glands of patients with Sjögren's syndrome. The appearance of sialectasis is sometimes referred to as a 'snow-storm effect'. The role of sialography in the diagnosis and management of tumours of the salivary glands is controversial and may well have been superseded by computed tomography with or without combined sialography. Sialography may still have a role to play in investigation of salivary swelling, since it can provide useful information whether a lesion is intraglandular or arising within adjacent tissues resulting in gland displacement.

Sialography is basically a safe and simple procedure, the only contra-indications being allergy to iodine or the presence of acute infection. It has been suggested that sialography does produce a bacteraemia, and therefore patients at risk from infective endocarditis should be given prophylactic antibiotics.

Scintiscanning

Radioisotopic study of salivary gland function is based on the ability of salivary glands to uptake radioisotopes selectively from the bloodstream. In practice, radioisotopes of iodine have too long a half-life to be useful clinically and therefore a related compound, technetium pertechnetate, which is handled like iodine by the major salivary gland, is used routinely. The isotope is introduced intravenously. The head and neck are scanned by techniques which pick up isotopic emissions and the major salivary glands are then visualized (Figure 18.4). The technique allows comparison of uptake in glands on the right with those on the left. Overall uptake can be quantified to detect generalized functional discrepancy.

Refinements of this basic technique involve the use of radioisotopes, such as selenomethionine and gallium, which are claimed to be selectively retained by certain salivary gland neoplasms.

Further reading

Lamey, P-J., Boyle, M. A., MacFarlane, T. W. and Samaranayake, L. P. (1987) Acute suppurative parotitis in outpatients: microbiologic and post-treatment sialographic findings. *Oral Surgery, Oral Medicine, Oral Pathology*, **63**, 37–41

Lamey, P-J., Lewis, M. A. O., Crawford, D. J. and MacDonald, D. G. (1989) Necrotising sialometaplasia presenting as greater palatine nerve anaesthesia. *International Journal of Oral Maxillofacial Surgery*, **18**, 70–72

Lewis, M. A. O., Lamey, P-J., and Gibson, J. (1989) Quantitative bacteriology of a case of acute parotitis. *Oral Surgery, Oral Medicine, Oral Pathology*, **68**, 571–575

Lewis, M. A. O., Lamey, P-J., Strang, R. and Mason, W. (1990) Clinical application of continuous infusion pressure-monitored sialography. *Dento Facial Maxillo Facial Radiology*, **20**, 68–72

Lewis, M. A. O., MacFarlane, T. W., Lamey, P-J., Leishman, R. E. and Howie, N. M. (1993) Quantitative bacteriology of the parotid salivary gland in health and Sjögren's syndrome. *Microbial Ecology in Health and Disease*, **6**, 29–34

Luyk, N. H., Doyle, T. and Ferguson, M. M. (1991) Recent trends in imaging of the salivary gland. *Dentomaxillofacial Radiology*, **20**, 3–10

MacFarlane, T. W. and Samaranayake, L. P. (1989) *Clinical Oral Microbiology*, Wright, London

MacGregor, I. A. and McGregor, F. M. (1986) *Cancer of the Face and Mouth*, Churchill Livingstone, Edinburgh

Mandel, I. D. (1990) The diagnostic uses of saliva. *Journal of Oral Pathology and Medicine*, **19**, 119–125

Mason, D. K. and Chisholm, D. M. (1975) *Salivary Glands in Health and Disease*, W. B. Saunders, London

Millard, H. D. and Mason, D. K. (1989) *Perspectives on 1988 World Workshop on Oral Medicine*, Section V pp. 283–327, Year Book Publishers, London

Scully, C. (1986) Sjögren's syndrome: clinical and laboratory features, immunopathogenesis and management. *Oral Surgery, Oral Medicine, Oral Pathology*, **62**, 510–523

Thorn, J. J., Prause, J. U. and Oxholm, P. (1989) Sialochemistry in Sjögren's syndrome: a review. *Journal of Oral Pathology and Medicine*, **18**, 457–468

Part Seven
Prescribing for Oral Disease

Chapter 19
Prescribing

19.1 Availability of medicines

19.2 Prescription writing

19.3 Controlled drugs

19.4 Precautions in prescribing

19.5 Storage of drugs

19.1 Availability of medicines

The availability of medicines to the general public varies widely in different parts of the world. In the UK substances used as medicinal products are controlled by the Medicines Act (1968) and fall into three categories, depending on their availability to the patient.

1. General sales list (GSL) – substances which can be supplied without the need for prescription or presence of a pharmacist at the time of sale.
2. Pharmacy medicines (P) – substances which can be supplied without the need for prescription, but which do require a pharmacist to be present at the time of sale.
3. Prescription only medicine (POM) – substances which can only be supplied by a pharmacist on prescription by an appropriate practitioner.

Drug therapy should only be employed when it is thought to be an essential part of patient management, since any agent has the potential to produce adverse effects, which are sometimes life threatening. There are many potential drug interactions involving medicines which are used for the management of oral disease; examples of these are shown in Table 19.1. Therefore, care must be taken when selecting a medication, and guidance on interactions is available in the Dental Practitioners' Formulary (DPF).

Patient compliance with drug therapy for orofacial disease is likely to be poor once acute symptoms, especially pain, have subsided. It is essential to explain to the patient the nature and action of any drug prescribed.

19.2 Prescription writing

A prescription is the authority for a pharmacist to supply a patient with a specified drug regime (Figure 19.1). A number of rules in prescribing exist.

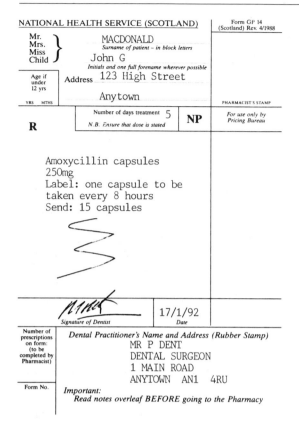

Figure 19.1 Prescription

1. The script must be in English and written in indelible ink or typewritten.
2. Apart from details of treatment the script should include:
   (a) the name, address and age of patient (if under 12 years);
   (b) the name, address and status of the practitioner issuing the prescription;
   (c) the date of issue and signature of the prescribing practitioner.
3. Details of treatment (abbreviations should be avoided):
   (a) number of days of treatment;
   (b) name of drug;
   (c) format of the drug;
   (d) strength of the drug (the use of decimal points should be avoided);
   (e) frequency of treatment;
   (f) special instructions;

(g) total amount of medicine to be dispensed;
(h) if the name of the drug should not appear on the label of the medicine, then NP should be deleted from this prescription.

Details of points (d) and (f) will be included on the label of the medicine. A prescription will be valid for 6 months from the date it is signed.

19.3 Controlled drugs

Regulations exist which limit the prescribing of controlled drugs. The prescription of drugs included in Schedules 1–5 as defined by the Misuse of Drugs Regulations has to comply with certain modification of details for prescription writing, listed above. Dental surgeons in the UK may store or prescribe drugs from Schedules 2, 3 and 4 as long as they are used solely for the purpose of dental treatment. Drugs included in these groups include (2) pethidine, morphine and dihydrocodeine, (3) pentazocine and (4) benzodiazepines.

The modifications for Schedules 2 and 3 are as follows:

1. The prescription, apart from the prescribed address, must be written in indelible ink.
2. Points (c), (d) and (g) above must be given in both words and figures.
3. The prescription should be endorsed 'for dental treatment only'.
4. The prescription should be signed and dated by the prescriber.

A register containing details of supply and dispensing *must* be kept for drugs specified in Schedules 1 and 2.

19.4 Precautions in prescribing
Children

Children differ from adults in their response to drugs and doses should therefore be adjusted accordingly. The formulary often provides information on the appropriate doses of individual drugs for children, usually based on body weight. Alternatively, adjustments may be made on the following age ranges: neonate (first month); infant (up to one year); 1–5 years and 6–12 years.

If recommended doses are not stated then the appropriate dose may be calculated using age, body weight or surface area. A reference guide to the percentage of adult doses based on these factors is provided in the formulary.

Elderly

Elderly patients require special consideration when prescribing, due to a number of factors including altered absorption, metabolism and excretion. Reduced renal clearance is especially important and can easily result in excessive levels of a drug in the body. It is therefore standard practice initially to prescribe 50% of the standard adult dose for elderly individuals. It is not uncommon for elderly individuals to be receiving multiple drugs and there is often therefore a potential for drug interactions. When prescribing for elderly patients it is especially important to state the taking or application of a medicament in clear, simple instructions.

Liver disease

The majority of drugs are principally metabolized in the liver and therefore the presence of liver disease may alter the response to any drug. Fortunately there is a large reserve of hepatic function and advanced disease has to be present before important changes occur. The formulary provides information on those drugs which should be used with caution in the presence of liver disease.

Renal impairment

Many drugs or their metabolites are excreted by the kidney and therefore reduced renal function may lead to toxic levels of drug within the body. Some drugs should be avoided in the presence of renal disease, whilst the dosages of others should be reduced.

Pregnancy and breast-feeding

Many drugs have the potential for inducing harmful effects on the development of the foetus at any stage of development. It is therefore sensible to limit prescribing to pregnant women to essential drugs only. The period of greatest risk in producing congenital malformations (teratogenic) is from the third to eleventh week of pregnancy.

Toxic effects of drugs can be produced by transfer of drug from mother to child through breast milk. Drug therapy should therefore be limited to essential drugs only during breast-feeding.

Drug interactions

Any potential drug interactions should be excluded prior to the prescribing of a particular agent. Information on interactions is available in the Practitioners Formulary. Some of the more common drug interactions occurring in dentistry are detailed in Table 19.1.

Adverse drug reactions

Any unwanted or unexpected effect of drug therapy should be reported to an appropriate authority. In the UK the Committee on Safety of Medicines (CSM) operates a confidential system (yellow card system) which can be used to register a suspected adverse drug event. The reporting dentist or doctor should provide details of the patient, the suspected drug therapy (including date started and date stopped) and the suspected reaction. In 1991 a total of 20 272 suspected adverse drug reactions were reported to the CSM which exceeded all previous years. This figure however is likely to be a gross underestimate since it is generally accepted that only 10% of even the most serious

Table 19.1 Examples of some drug interactions

Drug	Interacting drug	Effect	Comments
Penicillins	Probenecid	Blood antibiotic level elevated or prolonged	Effect used therapeutically for prophylaxis of endocarditis
	Oral contraceptives	Decreased effectiveness of contraceptive	Warn patient
Erythromycin	Carbamazepine	Increased blood levels with toxicity	Use with caution
	Coumarins	Potentiated anticoagulant effect	Avoid if possible
Metronidazole	Alcohol	'Antabuse' like action	Patient should avoid alcohol
	Coumarins	Potentiated anticoagulant effect	Avoid if possible
	Phenytoin	Increased blood levels with toxic effects	Inform medical practitioner
Tetracycline	Oral contraceptives	Decreased effectiveness of contraceptive	Warn patient
Hydrocortisone	Oral hypoglycaemics	Reduce hypoglycaemic effect	Avoid if possible
Aspirin	Coumarins	Potentiated anticoagulant effect	Avoid if possible

adverse reactions are reported. All clinicians are encouraged to report suspected reactions to ensure safe prescribing.

Oral side-effects of drug therapy include xerostomia, lichenoid reactions and oral candidiosis. The presentation and management of such reactions is discussed elsewhere in this text.

19.5 Storage of drugs

Drugs stored in surgeries or clinics should be kept in appropriate secure cupboards. Special regulations apply to the storage of all controlled drugs as defined by Misuse of Drugs (Safe Custody) Regulations 1973 (amended 1985).

Further reading

Dental Practitioners' Formulary 1992–1994, British Dental Association, British Medical Association and Pharmaceutical Society of Great Britain, London

Duxbury, A. J., Leach, F. N., Duxbury, J. T. (1984) Common prescribing problems. *Dental Update*, **11** 101–110

Walton, J. G., Thompson, J. W. and Seymour, R. A. (1989) *Textbook of Dental Pharmacology and Therapeutics*, Oxford University Press, Oxford

Part Eight

Medical Emergencies

Chapter 20
Medical emergencies

A life-threatening medical emergency can occur at any time or in any place. Fortunately medical emergencies in the dental surgery are rare and when fatalities have ensued they have been associated with the provision of a general anaesthetic. The performance of general anaesthesia and sedation in dental surgeries in the UK has recently undergone review, and strict recommendations on the training of the medical staff involved and the type of equipment available have been made. There is a potential, however, for medical emergencies to occur in the dental surgery regardless of the involvement of anaesthesia. This is especially true for those acute conditions which may be precipitated by anxiety, because undergoing dental treatment is a stressful event for many patients. The dental team should therefore be capable of providing basic management of the range of medical emergencies which may occur. This can be achieved by ensuring that all members of the practice staff receive appropriate training, in particular in how to clear and maintain the airway and how to provide cardiopulmonary resuscitation (CPR).

20.1 Faint (syncope)

Fainting reportedly occurs in approximately 2% of patients undergoing extractions under local anaesthesia and is the most common cause of loss of consciousness in the dental surgery. The mechanism of fainting is not fully understood, but in the dental surgery it is likely to involve an emotional episode (anxiety or pain) which initially induces a rise in blood pressure and tachycardia. This in turn produces a parasympathetic (vagal) response, with dilation of vessels in the skeletal muscle, a fall in blood pressure and bradycardia.

Signs

Dizziness, nausea, clammy skin are all signs that the patient may faint. The pulse is first slow and weak, then becomes rapid and full.

Management

The patient should be laid supine, with the legs raised and clothing loosened.

Recovery should be rapid, but if it is delayed atropine (0.5 mg) can be administered intramuscularly.

20.2 Hypoglycaemia

Patients with insulin-dependent diabetes who either take an excessive amount of insulin or do not eat at the correct time may lose consciousness due to hypoglycaemia.

Signs

Signs of hypoglycaemia include mental confusion, irritability, sweating and a full and rapid pulse.

Management

The patient is laid flat. If the patient is conscious, 50 g of glucose is given orally. If he or she is unconscious either 20–50 ml of 50% glucose is given as an intravenous infusion or 1 mg glucagon is given intramuscularly or subcutaneously. An ambulance should be called. Recovery should be rapid.

20.3 Steroid collapse

Any patient who has a history of previous systemic corticosteroid therapy has the potential for fatal circulatory collapse due to adrenocortical suppression if stressed. It is generally accepted that any history of corticosteroid therapy in the preceding 2 years requires a prophylactic corticosteroid regime. It is recommended that 100 mg of hydrocortisone should be given intravenously prior to any stressful procedure, such as extractions or minor oral surgery under local anaesthesia.

Further hydrocortisone (100–500 mg) should be given if a patient shows any signs of circulatory collapse during operation. If collapse occurs the patient should be given oxygen and an ambulance summoned.

20.4 Anaphylaxis

Anaphylactic shock represents an immediate (type I) hypersensitivity reaction involving the release of large quantities of histamine that produce bronchospasm and a drop in blood pressure. Although anaphylaxis is a rare occurrence in the dental surgery, it is a well-recognized complication of systemic administration of penicillin and, occasionally, local anaesthetics. Reactions to penicillin may either occur within 30 seconds of a penicillin injection or within 30 minutes of oral administration of the drug.

Signs

Signs include facial oedema, urticarial rash, pallor, sweating, cold clammy skin, a rapid and weak pulse and wheezing.

Management

The patient is laid flat and given 1 ml of 1:1000 adrenaline intramuscularly, then 200 mg of hydrocortisone sodium succinate intravenously. Oxygen is administered and an ambulance called.

20.5 Epilepsy

Although the development of anticonvulsant drugs has resulted in effective prophylaxis of epileptic seizures, some patients may suffer a major fit in the dental surgery.

Signs

Signs include loss of consciousness, generalized muscular contraction (chronic stage), uncontrolled jerking of the body (chronic stage) and incontinence.

Management

All equipment should be removed from the patient's immediate environment. If convulsions do not stop within 5 minutes, 10 mg diazepam is given intravenously. An ambulance should be called.

20.6 Angina and myocardial infarction

Angina literally means tightness, but the term 'angina pectoris' is widely used to describe the symptoms associated with myocardial ischaemia.

Signs of angina

Retrosternal pain radiating down the left arm.

Management of angina

The patient should rest. Glyceryl trinitrate is given sublingually. The pain should subside with rest.

Myocardial ischaemia may be due to myocardial infarction which produces severe and prolonged pain.

Signs of myocardial ischaemia

Severe crushing retrosternal pain radiating down the left arm, nausea, cold, clammy skin, pallor and a weak pulse.

Management of myocardial ischaemia

The patient should be reassured, oxygen (with or without 50% nitrous oxide) is administered and pethidine, 25–50 mg, given intravenously. An ambulance should be called.

20.7 Cardiac arrest

Cardiac arrest may occur in the dental surgery for a number of reasons, including myocardial infarction, sensitivity to drugs or hypoxia occurring during general anaesthesia.

Signs

Signs include loss of consciousness, absent pulse, cyanosis and dilated pupils.

Management

Help should be summoned, and the patient laid flat on the floor. Two sharp blows should be given to midsternum. The airway is cleared, and the head placed back with the mandible up. Ventilation is provided either by the expired air method (+ Brook airway); or by the mechanical method using an Ambu bag or Air Viber bag with oropharyngeal airway. The circulation is restored by cardiac massage. An ambulance should be called.

20.8 Cerebrovascular accident (CVA, stroke)

A stroke may be of slow or sudden onset and there are varying degrees of severity. Cerebral infarction (thrombosis 90%, embolism 10%) accounts for most strokes. There is a potential for a stroke to occur within the dental surgery, especially in elderly patients. Approximately 25% of victims die as a result of the first stroke.

Signs

Signs include loss of consciousness, limb weakness, speech defect and vomiting.

Management

The patient is positioned upright, oxygen is provided and an ambulance called.

Table 20.1 Suggested basic emergency kit for dental surgery

Equipment	Drugs
Ambu bag	Adrenaline injection (1:1000)
Brook airway	1 ml ampoules
Guedel oropharyngeal airway	Hydrocortisone sodium succinate (100 mg)
Aspirator tips	Glucose powder, 50 g for one drink
Tourniquet	Glucose intravenous infusion
Disposable syringes	50% solution in 50 ml ampoule
Needles/butterflies	Glucagon (1 mg)
	Chlorpheniramine (10 mg/ml)
	Diazepam injection (5 mg/ml)

A supply of oxygen should be readily available

20.9 Medical emergency kit

A suitable kit containing a selection of equipment and medications should be available in the surgery. The minimum contents of an emergency kit are outlined in Table 20.1. Emergency kits are available commercially, but some practitioners prefer to make their own kit up. However the kit is made up, it is essential that stocks are maintained and replaced when expiry dates are passed.

Further reading

Edmondson, H. D. and Frame, J. W. (1986) Medical emergencies in general practice 1. Acute medical problems. *Dental Update*, **13**, 211–220

Edmondson, H. D. and Frame, J. W. (1986) Medical emergencies in general practice 1. Cardiopulmonary emergencies. *Dental Update*, **13**, 263–273

Scully, C. (1988) Management of emergencies. In *Clinical Dentistry in Health and Disease*, volume 1, *The Dental Patient*, (ed. C. Scully), Butterworth-Heinemann, Oxford, pp 104–116

Appendix

Infective endocarditis and dental treatment

Dental procedures which cause a bacteraemia (1) may lead to the development of infective endocarditis in certain risk patients (2). Antibiotic therapy should be provided as prophylaxis to prevent the endocarditis (3). Additional measures should also be undertaken (4).

1. (a) Dental procedures known to produce a significant bacteraemia
   Tooth extraction
   Subgingival periodontal procedures
   Periodontal surgery
   (b) Dental procedures which may produce a significant bacteraemia
   Incision of an acute dentoalveolar abscess
   Re-implantation of a tooth
   Repositioning of a displaced tooth
   Endodontic therapy involving periapical tissues
   Sialography
2. 'Risk' factors likely to predispose a patient to infective endocarditis
   Rheumatic valve disease
   Congenital heart defect
   Other heart valve disease (including murmur)
   Heart valve surgery
   Prosthetic heart valves
   Cardiac surgery (some)
   Previous infective endocarditis
3. Suggested antibiotic prophylaxis for endocarditis (adapted from the recommendation of the Endocarditis Working Party of the British Society for Antimicrobial Chemotherapy (1992). *Lancet*, **339**).

(i) *Dental procedures under local or no anaesthesia*
   For patients not allergic to penicillin and not prescribed penicillin more than once in the previous month (excluding those with history of previous endocarditis):
   Amoxycillin
   Adults: 3 g single oral dose taken under supervision one hour before dental procedure
   Children under 10 years old: half adult dose
   Children under 5 years old: quarter adult dose
   or
   For patients allergic to penicillin or prescribed penicillin more than once in the previous month (excluding those with history of previous endocarditis):
   Clindamycin
   Adults: 600 mg single oral dose taken under supervision one hour before dental procedure
   Children under 10 years old: half adult dose
   Children under 5 years old: quarter adult dose

(ii) *Under general anaesthesia*
   (c) For patients not allergic to penicillin and not given penicillin more than once in the previous month:
   Amoxycillin
   Adults: 1 g intramuscularly of intravenously just before induction, plus 500 mg by mouth 6 hours later
   Children under 10 years old: half adult dose
   or

Amoxycillin

Adults: 3 g oral dose 4 hours before anaesthesia, followed by a further 3 g by mouth as soon as possible after operation

Children under 10 years old: half adult dose

Children under 5 years old: quarter adult dose

or

Amoxycillin and probenecid

Adults: amoxycillin 3 g together with probenecid 1 g orally 4 hours before operation

(d) Patients who are allergic to penicillin and require a general anaesthetic should be referred to hospital.

4. Additional measures for prophylaxis of endocarditis

Irrigation of gingival margins or surgical site prior to procedure with antiseptic.

Advise patient to report immediately any unexplained illness, however mild, in the subsequent 2 months.

Suggest the patient carries a warning card giving details of his or her heart specialist who could be contacted for advice on management (cards are available free from British Heart Foundation, 14 Fitzhardinge Street, London W1H 4DH).

Ensure that the patient maintains good oral hygiene.

Index